D0504805

Award-winning writer, television broadcaster and author of numerous bestsellers, **Leslie Kenton** is described by the press as 'the guru of health and fitness' and 'the most original voice in health'. A shining example of energy and commitment, she is highly respected for her thorough reporting. Leslie was born in California, and is the daughter of jazz musician Stan Kenton. After leaving Stanford University she journeyed to Europe in her early twenties, settling first in Paris, then in Britain where she has since remained. She has raised four children on her own by working as a television broadcaster, novelist, writer and teacher on health and for fourteen years she was an editor at *Harpers & Queen*.

Leslie's writing on mainstream health is internationally known and has appeared in *Vogue*, the *Sunday Times*, *Cosmopolitan*, and the *Daily Mail*. She is the author of many health books and recently she turned to fiction with *Ludwig* – her first novel. Former consultant to a medical corporation in the USA and to the Open University's Centre of Continuing Education, Leslie's writing has won several awards including the PPA 'Technical Writer of the Year'. Her work was honoured by her being asked to deliver the McCarrison Lecture at the Royal Society of Medicine.

Russell Cronin worked as a cook in London and New York before he started writing, mostly about food and drink, for *Arena* magazine. He created an innovative weekly food and drink gossip, called 'Gastropod', which ran in *The Independent* for two and a half years and, in conjunction with wagamama noodle bar, wrote a recipe book with elements of philosophy, called *Way of the Noodle*. It was while working with wagamama that Russell first read Leslie Kenton's *Raw Energy* and began experimenting with freshly-extracted raw juices. He set up and ran what is probably the country's first travelling juice bar at the 25th Glastonbury Festival in 1995 and is now developing the juice bar concept with The Fresh Juice Company.

JUICE HIGH

Leslie Kenton
with Russell Cronin

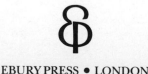

EBURY PRESS • LONDON

To all those who seek the highs
but are devastated by the lows
that usually follow
this little book is dedicated

1 3 5 7 9 10 8 6 4 2

Text copyright © Leslie Kenton and Russell Cronin 1996

The right of Leslie Kenton and Russell Cronin to be identified as the
authors of this book has been asserted by them in accordance with the
Copyright, Designs and Patents Act, 1988.

First published in the United Kingdom in 1996 by
Ebury Press
Random House
20 Vauxhall Bridge Road
London SW1V 2SA

Random House Australia (Pty) Limited
20 Alfred Street, Milsons Point, Sydney,
New South Wales 2061, Australia

Random House New Zealand Limited
18 Poland Road, Glenfield,
Auckland 10, New Zealand

Random House South Africa (Pty) Limited
PO BOX 337, Bergvlei, South Africa

Random House Canada
1265 Aerowood Drive, Mississauga
Ontario L4W 1B9, Canada

Random House UK Limited Reg. No. 954009

A CIP catalogue record for this book is available
from the British Library

ISBN: 0 09 182002 2

Printed and bound in Great Britain by
Mackays of Chatham plc, Kent

Papers used by Ebury Press are natural, recyclable products made
from wood grown in sustainable forests.

Contents

Authors' Note

The material in this book is intended for information purposes only. None of the suggestions or information is meant in any way to be prescriptive. Any attempt to treat a medical condition should always come under the direction of a competent physician – and neither we nor the publisher can accept responsibility for injuries or illness arising out of a failure by a reader to take medical advice. We are only reporters. We also have a profound interest in helping ourselves and others to maximise potentials for positive health which include being able to live at a high level of energy, intelligence and creativity. For all three are expressions of harmony within a living, organic system.

Leslie Kenton
Russell Cronin
1996

Chapter One
Lifepower

As soon as you begin to incorporate freshly-extracted, raw vegetable and fruit juices into your lifestyle, something amazing starts happening to you. First you will notice the terrific lift that just one glass of fresh juice can give you, particularly when taken first thing on an empty stomach. Imagine what life might be like if, instead of trying to kick-start yourself with strong coffee in the mornings, you could drink a glass of raw juice and almost immediately feel refreshed, alert and eager to see what another day has in store. This is the liberating effect of the Juice High.

Raw juice is the most perfect fuel for your body. Its high water content means that it is easily assimilated and tends to cleanse and nurture the body while supplying it with a full range of essential nutrients. That's all there is to it. Except, of course, that raw juice also has another property, a mysterious factor X, which scientists have yet to properly understand. Freshly-extracted juices are bursting with *Lifepower* – a natural, raw energy that is miraculous in its beneficial effect on the human body.

The nutritional and recuperative value of raw juice has been well known to doctors and natural health practitioners since the turn of the century, when several of the most eminent pioneers in the field started experimenting with raw foods to improve their own health. The famous **Rohsäft Kur** (raw juice cure) developed by Dr Max Bircher-Benner and Dr Max Gerson nearly ninety years ago is now acknowledged to be the single most potent short-term antidote to fatigue and stress. Until recently it's been the preserve of the privileged few who could afford to go to an exclusive health spa.

Now, with the advent of affordable domestic centrifugal juice extractors, hi-tech nutrition and the salvation of raw juice is within reach. Our raw juice cure – the Juice Blitz (see Chapter 3) – can be undertaken over a weekend in the comfort of your own home. It can be used as a quick-fix detox programme, or as the first step towards changing your life.

Raw Energy Rush

Energy is the essence of life, the force that makes everything feasible and achievable. In the body, energy is produced by billions of tiny powerhouses – or cells – and for our bodies to function at peak efficiency, we must provide the optimum conditions for each cell to do its work. In order to be fit and healthy and to live a long and active life, we need plenty of fresh air and the vital nourishment that comes from eating whole foods.

Only in comparatively recent times has mankind come to realise that the condition of the human body is inextricably bound up with the quality of the food we ingest and the air we breathe. Over the past hundred years, since the Industrial Revolution, the quality of both our food and air and consequently our ability to be healthy has declined dramatically. Because we now live in an environment that is increasingly toxic, we need the most effective form of nutrition in order to combat its degenerative effects and to revitalise our bodies.

Not only do our bodies need the full range of essential nutrients to be healthy, but they need them to be available in the form in which they can most readily be utilised. That means *in the raw*. Raw fruits and vegetables contain the most valuable array of vitamins, minerals and amino acids, but they also have a uniquely healthful quality which science has yet to decode. Since scientists cannot formulate into pills nutrients they haven't yet identified, the biggest synthetic vitamin pill you can buy can never compensate for a lack of the natural goodness that is only contained within raw fruits and vegetables.

The simple reason why raw juices are so beneficial is because they deliver, straight into your system, the most complete range of nutrients in their most vital form, suspended in water from an organic source and brimming with enzymes. Enzymes are the intangible living elements which act as the catalyst for innumerable chemical reactions within the body, promoting efficient assimilation and enabling the metabolic processes that support high levels of energy and promote good health.

Good health should not be defined as the absence of disease, but as a vital, dynamic condition in which we feel positively charged and fully able to take whatever life has to throw at us. This is the property we call Raw Energy and the most immediate way to experience its Lifepower is by drinking raw juice.

Re: Juice

Replenishment is the immutable law of life. If we fail to replace the water in our bodies that is lost through perspiration, we become dehydrated and soon start to wilt. The soft drinks industry is a big and rapidly growing business that churns out billions of bucks' worth of propaganda to persuade us that cans of carbonated syrup will satisfy our thirst and enhance our energy. There's even a breed of so-called 'sports drinks' which are claimed not only to replace bodily fluids, but also to reinvigorate tired muscles. Actually, the last thing most of these synthetic products can offer your body is proper refreshment and, while they may give you a sugar shock or a caffeine jolt, as a source of prolonged energy they are worthless.

In fact, the kind of water your body craves and depends upon to function at peak efficiency does not come out of a tap, or from a bottle, but is only found in fresh fruits and vegetables. Your body can't use the water in fizzy drinks, or beer, and so those fluids pass quickly through to the bladder. The water extracted from raw fruit and vegetables, however, has a unique organic quality and is readily absorbed by the body. Because it is so rich in essential micro-nutrients, raw juice effectively replenishes lost energy. In fact, raw juice is the most profoundly refreshing fluid you can drink.

Fatal Fizz

People working in the soul-sapping environment of, say, a modern office building will reach for coffee and fizzy drinks in the middle of the afternoon in the hope that it will give them enough mental energy to make it through to the end of another hectic day. Then they experience a corresponding energy slump on the way home, arriving irritable and exhausted and good for nothing but going early to bed. The end result of living like this is a kind of chronic fatigue that often manifests itself as indifferent, fatalistic lethargy.

So-called 'soft drinks' bring nutritionally empty calories into your body which you can ill afford. A twelve ounce can of cola contains seven teaspoons (40 g) of sugar and is full of chemicals that pollute your body, including phosphoric acid – the chemical used to etch glass – which impedes the function of the kidneys and leaches calcium from bones, teeth and hair. As for the 'diet' varieties, quite apart from the proven fact that drinking them will do absolutely nothing to help you lose weight, they are an even more noxious cocktail of artificial chemicals. Stay away from them.

But the main reason you will want to abandon soft drinks and make raw juice your preferred beverage is because it tastes fantastic. If you've tried bottled carrot juice and didn't like it, don't be put off from tasting the real thing. Freshly-extracted carrot juice is sweet, creamy and delicious. Mix it with apple juice and you have a whole drink that is perfectly balanced for your nutritional needs, but also tastes so good that we have never come across anyone who doesn't like it.

Pure Fuel

All our energy is ultimately derived from the food we eat and without proper digestion there can be no such thing as good nutrition. Food passes through the body, from the oesophagus via the stomach and gastro-intestinal tract, where it is broken down and nutrients are assimilated into the body. Although it's true that we are what we eat, it's more accurate to say that we are what we assimilate. By extracting the juices of fruits and vegetables, removing their fibre, we can provide the body with an excellent source of nutrition that is virtual-ly pre-digested, so that it is assimilated with minimum effort.

No less important than efficient assimilation is the prompt elimination of food wastes that will otherwise accumulate in the colon and decay, breeding putre-factive bacteria that release toxins which get into the bloodstream, spreading all sorts of sickness throughout the body. The residues of digested food pass from the small intestine into the colon in liquid form and are moved along by the action of peristalsis, to be eliminat-ed from the bowels. The fibres in raw foods assist this process, acting as a kind of intestinal broom, but when food is denatured by processing, the action is more like a filthy mop that leaves a trail of slime coating the intestinal walls and making the colon sluggish and slow.

There is nothing in raw juice that your body cannot use and, therefore, nothing that it need work to expel. Instead, the body can concentrate on getting rid of old waste and the action of raw juice will encourage that by irrigating the intestine and causing a chain reaction in the colon that can have explosive results! This laxative effect, which is particularly pronounced with fruit juices, is highly beneficial because it helps the body to detoxify itself, providing the ideal environment for biological regeneration.

Rejuvenation

As you become accustomed to juicing, and to the effect of raw juice on your bowel movements, you may well shed excess weight. As your colon cleanses itself and your metabolism becomes more efficient, and so long as you are not continually clogging your system with junk foods, the body will revert to its natural weight. You start to feel fitter and younger than you have in years and you get used to old friends telling you how well you look. What's more, when you see yourself in the mirror, you even *look* younger; your complexion seems smoother and wrinkles recede. This is no illusion. The Lifepower of freshly-extracted juices has the potential to rejuvenate your body in a way that quite literally makes you younger.

What makes us old is not merely the passing years but environmental poisons, inadequate food and mental stress. These factors conspire to cause an acidic chemical imbalance within the body that is redressed by raw juice, which tends to be alkaline. One of the most significant factors in premature ageing is the effect of free radical particles in atmospheric pollution, biochemical bully boys that vandalise our bodies at a cellular level. The best way to combat them is with a regular intake of raw juice.

Smog Off

The infernal internal combustion engine has proved to be the most destructive invention of the twentieth century and it's going to be difficult to explain to future generations why we allowed their air to be poisoned by exhaust fumes and condemned them to grow up with a range of respiratory illnesses caused by pollution. Just breathe in by the side of the road and savour that acrid cocktail of sulphur dioxide and carbon monoxide, liberally laced with benzene and hydrocarbons.

Your body is a biochemical battleground in which the baddies are the free radicals that are particularly prevalent in car exhaust fumes. Scientifically, free radicals are molecules with an unpaired electron, which makes them highly reactive and inclined to stabilise themselves by attracting another electron from any other molecule, particularly the lipids in cell membranes. These are the fundamental building blocks of our bodily tissues. By knocking out a few of these blocks in a process called 'lipid peroxidation', free radicals can bring the whole lot tumbling down by causing an ever-amplifying series of chain reactions that leads to the destruction of tissues. That's how smoking and breathing heavily-polluted air corrodes our vitality, causes cancer and makes us old before our time.

Still, what can you do? Walking around in a hi-tech gas mask is hardly practicable, so you'd better ensure you get yourself a plentiful supply of the fresh vitamins that can prevent or retard free radical damage. You need plenty of A, C and E, the so-called anti-oxidant vitamins, as well as other recently-discovered plant-based anti-oxidant compounds that are found only in fresh fruit and vegetables, to protect yourself against the degenerative effects of pollution. The best way to ensure an adequate supply is . . . to drink plenty of freshly-extracted raw juice.

Food Glut

A potentially catastrophic revolution has taken place in our eating habits over the past century. Commercial considerations, rather than concern for human health, have been allowed to dictate the way in which our food is produced, processed and distributed. Crops are grown

13

in chemically-fertilised soils, doused with pesticides and then made into products which are packaged to be shipped over long distances and stored for extended periods. All these complicated modern practices conspire to destroy the wholesome quality of the foodstuffs we can most easily afford to buy from the local supermarket.

The convenience foods that dominate the diets of most of us privileged to be living in the affluent, developed world have had their nutritional integrity destroyed. Their natural goodness has been systematically stripped from them and replaced with a range of artificial additives to enhance their taste and mouthfeel and to prolong their shelf life as far as possible. Refined foods are loaded with excessive amounts of fats and sugars, but offer the body practically nothing in terms of nutrition, failing adequately to satisfy our appetite for real food and tempting us to overeat, compulsively.

Fat Chances

Widespread obesity is a relatively new phenomenon, but one which is now a contributing factor in a range of chronic degenerative diseases that have become the biggest killers of modern times: cardiovascular conditions and cancer. While it is possible to subsist on a diet of microwavable ready meals, it's impossible to thrive. Despite the miracles of medical science, statistics demonstrate that the population as a whole is not getting healthier.

A poor diet undermines good health and leaves you in poor shape to cope with the stresses and strains of modern life but, much worse, it's bad for the soul. The physiological effect of a high-gunk diet – that's one that tends to clog your system with rubbish that's nutritionally worthless and hard to digest – is to slow you down, making you feel heavy. Psychologically, that can only make you depressed.

Stop Wilting

Before World War II all crops were grown without the use of chemicals, which is to say organically. The organic matter in healthy soil creates fertility and promotes the growth of strong, healthy plants. Artificial chemicals interfere with that vital process, stripping the soil of its natural goodness and depriving the plants grown in it of essential minerals and other micro-substances. Destroy the soil's organic matter through chemical farming, and slowly, but inexorably, the health of people and animals that live on the foods grown in it will be undermined and their resistance to disease will be compromised.

The body has an amazing ability to compensate for missing nutrients, but after years of eating nutritionally depleted foods, widespread deficiencies are becoming apparent and all sorts of metabolic distortions follow. Being fat is the most obvious one, but perhaps the most insidious effect of the modern diet is the imbalance of sodium and potassium in many people's bodies.

Sodium and potassium are nutritional antagonists that act synergistically in the body to regulate the osmotic pressure on the walls of each cell. When properly balanced, these two minerals also transmit electrochemical impulses throughout the body, keeping the whole organism vibrant. Too much sodium or too little potassium and the organism starts to wilt, causing the kind of chronic fatigue that has you reaching for coffee and chocolate biscuits in the middle of the afternoon just to keep going.

That is what's happening to masses of people nowadays who have too much salt in their diet, promoting acidity in the body and undermining its resilience. What they need is potassium and the best way to get it – you've guessed it – is by drinking raw juice.

15

Get Smart

There's nothing controversial in the suggestion that eating fresh fruit and vegetables will significantly reduce your chances of dying prematurely from heart disease or cancer. The World Health Organisation recommends that we eat at least half a kilo of fresh fruit and vegetables every day. When the Europe Against Cancer campaign launched its 'Five-A-Day' initiative, aimed at encouraging the daily intake of at least five hundred-gramme portions of fruit and vegetables, they pointed out that Britain falls far short of the target, with the lowest fruit and vegetable consumption – and the highest incidence of heart disease – in Europe.

It's not just adults who require the raw energy of fresh foods to thrive. Unborn babies are particularly vulnerable: thousands have been born with spina bifida because their mothers were deficient in folic acid during the first six weeks of pregnancy, perhaps before many of them even realised they were pregnant. Folic acid is a soluble vitamin, a member of the B complex, which assists the formation of DNA. It's abundant in green vegetables like broccoli, but is easily destroyed by cooking.

Many children refuse to eat enough fresh vegetables because they say they don't like the taste. Sadly, many kids these days are addicted to sugar and so used to sloppy convenience foods that they can't be bothered to chew whole food properly. But fresh juices are easy to drink and it's no problem to persuade children to take them, since they taste delicious.

Get Juicing

Never forget that the body and mind are not separate entities, but are completely interdependent. The foods we consume dictate not only our physical well-being, but our moods and ability to think clearly. People who are in control of their health are in control of their destiny, able to work harder and more effectively to fulfil their dreams.

Once you start to incorporate freshly-extracted raw fruits and vegetable juices into your diet you will begin to arrest the build-up of toxins in your body. As you continue to take raw juices on a regular basis, the deadly degenerative effects of a junk diet will be reversed. This process of detoxification may be gradual or it may be quite dramatic, depending on the enthusiasm with which you take to raw juice, but its effects are always remarkable.

Raw juice will help you to build the stamina to cope with the debilitating stresses of modern life, but it can also transform the way you see the world around you. As your body re-balances itself, you'll find that your moods stabilise, too. Trivialities cease to upset you and you are able to keep things in perspective. Detoxifying the system and flushing your colon with raw juice actually helps you to think more clearly and rationally, to concentrate for longer and maintain a more optimistic frame of mind. This is the state we call Juice High and, unlike the high you get from coffee, or drugs, it is perfectly possible to stay high on raw juice all of the time.

Drinking raw juice is not like doing drugs. Drug users often say they are seeking enlightenment, to 'expand their minds', but by artificially altering their perceptions with chemicals they may be doing themselves damage. Whether or not drugs do long-term harm, their effects are temporary and usually followed by a 'crash' when the drug wears off. (Drinking raw juice, by the way, is the best possible thing you can do to recover from the after-effects of drug abuse or excessive drinking.) People take drugs to get 'out of it' and 'off their heads' but raw juice will have the opposite effect, making you feel more 'normal', better 'centred', and properly 'connected'.

Any raw juice is better than none at all, but if you use your juice well, and take it on a daily basis, you might just come to realise that, since you started juicing, not only has your health perked up, you feel positively happy.

Chapter Two
Get Juiced

Harmony is the underlying principle of life. All illnesses can be regarded as a manifestation of disharmony within the human body.

If all the metabolic processes that animate your body and enable you to live a fully active and healthy life are to work properly, the internal environment of the body requires perfect harmony. Breathing polluted air and eating processed foods replete with sugar, junk fats and refined carbohydrates (not to mention bad habits like drinking and smoking) conspire to create excess acidity and create a chemical imbalance within the body. All raw juices have a strongly alkalinising effect, tipping the pH balance back to normal, helping to restore harmony and enabling the body to cleanse and heal itself.

Juice It

There are three clearly defined stages in the body's utilisation of food: appropriation (eating and digestion); assimilation (taking in nutrients) and elimination (expelling waste products). While all these activities are always taking place to some extent, the function of each is heightened at different times during the course of a day. If you've ever slumped on the sofa after a big meal, unable to move, you'll know how much energy the process of breaking down food in the stomach requires. If you really stuff yourself, your body is forced to close down some of your other physiological functions while it gets to grips with digesting.

Because it requires so much energy, the body prefers to do most of the hard work of assimilation at night, while you sleep. By the time you wake up in the morning, you will have moved into the elimination cycle. This is not a matter of having a single bowel movement before breakfast, but a deep and thorough cleansing at cellular level, with wastes being expelled via all the organs of elimination, including the skin and lungs as well as the bowels and urinary tract. The elimination cycle lasts throughout the morning and that is the best time to take raw juices, particularly those freshly extracted from fruit.

Fruit juices are great for getting you moving in the mornings. All fruit contains fructose, the natural sugar that your body can use for fuel, and is usually around 90 per cent water, promoting prompt elimination. When perfectly ripe, fruit also contains its own digestive enzymes and is therefore virtually pre-digested – it passes rapidly through the stomach and into the intestines. Of course, fruit juices can cause a rapid rise in blood sugar, so diabetics and people who are prone to yeast infections should be careful how they use them, but most people will find the effect of a glass of raw fruit juice for breakfast quite invigorating. Drink a glass of freshly extracted watermelon, or pineapple, or pink grapefruit juice on an empty stomach and within fifteen minutes you'll be wide awake and ready to rock.

It is always best to take fruits or their juices on an empty stomach, since they cannot be so effective if their passage through the stomach is impeded by undigested food. In fact, resolving to consume nothing but raw juices and fruit from the moment you get up until lunchtime could well be the healthiest lifestyle decision you ever make. As the day progresses, incorporate more and more vegetables into your juices and switch their emphasis from sweet to savoury.

The Juice Kitchen

Undoubtedly the most useful tool in the juice kitchen is a vegetable peeler. Not a blunt old potato peeler, but a speed peeler with a pivoting head which can be bought from any catering supply shop if you can't find one in the local hardware store. Not all vegetables should be peeled, however, as their nutrients tend to be concentrated in the skin. Organic carrots, beetroots and apples are great juiced whole. Buy a scrubbing brush such as a nail brush to scrub the dirt off root vegetables. The brush will also be useful for scrubbing the strainer basket of your juicer.

Second, you need a sharp knife and a cutting board. If your chosen juicer has a spout rather than an integral jug, find some glasses that fit snugly under the spout, but buy an accurate measuring jug as well and use it to formulate your own recipes. Juicing directly into the glass saves on washing up, but it's useful to have a swizzle stick – a chop-stick will do – or a thin wooden spoon to stir your juices before serving.

Third, of course, you need a juicer – and it really does have to be more sophisticated than the traditional hand-held push-down-and-turn conical object at the back of your kitchen cupboard.

Buying a Juicer

Centrifugal juice extractors contain a basket, usually made from stainless steel, with sharp shredding blades at the bottom and a fine mesh screen at the sides. When you push fruit and vegetables through the rotating blades, the pulp is spun off into a receptacle at the back of the machine and the juice strained out through a spout, or into an integral jug. A juicer with a spout is better than one with a jug because then you can juice directly into a glass and there's less to wash up.

As with any domestic appliance, look for the most robust model you can get for your money. This means the one with the strongest motor and the strongest locking mechanism. Beware of two-speed juicers and those models with a hopper that simply clicks into place without your having to clamp it down. These rinky-dink features just give you more to go wrong.

One other thing to check before buying yo___
the size of the hole you are supposed to put the___
through. Some are really too small and it's a ___
have to slice even the skinniest carrot lengthways. ___

Russell once took a burned-out juicer back to the
shop when it was less than a year old and the salesman
asked how much he had used it. Actually, he'd used it
every day, but what was it designed for? Don't be afraid
to demand a demonstration of the model you intend to
buy, listen to the whine the motor makes and ask yourself if it sounds as if it can stand up to the job.

For details of other equipment, see Resources, page
147.

Next to Godliness

Cleanliness is important with regard to the proper
maintenance of your juicer, which will quickly become
stained unless you take proper care of it. The strong
natural pigments of the raw foods you'll be juicing will
inevitably stain the plastic parts of your juicer, so that
you will have to soak them regularly in a bleach solution
to keep your machine pristine. More importantly, you
must thoroughly scour your juicer every time you use it
with plenty of hot water, ensuring that the steel basket
that does the work of shredding is absolutely clean and
that there are no bits of vegetable matter caught in the
fine mesh of the sieve.

It's always easier to clean your juicer straight after
you've used it than it will be the next time you want to
use it. We find that it's good practice to clean the juicer
before drinking the juice we've just made. That way,
we're so eager to get the chore over with that the work
takes only a minute.

Get Freshness

Freshness is the first principle of good juicing. When buying fresh produce, don't let yourself be palmed off with

overripe fruit that's started to 'turn', or soft and sad-looking vegetables with limp leaves. Choose only the most perfectly ripe fruits and vegetables and don't buy more than you can use over a couple of days. You will be getting through a lot of produce, but don't be tempted to buy in bulk unless you're sure you're going to use it up. While it's often not necessary to peel the produce you'll be juicing, it *is* essential to wash it thoroughly, using a scrubbing brush if necessary, under cold running water.

Freshly-extracted juices must be drunk as soon as they are made, before their Raw Energy expires. The nutrients in raw juice are highly volatile and will begin to deteriorate as soon as they are in contact with fresh air, so that its essential vitality is quickly lost. If you want to demonstrate this for yourself, leave a glass of raw juice to stand for just a few minutes and you'll see how quickly it separates into a clear liquid (water) with a scummy head on top. A lot less inviting than the vividly coloured fluid you started with. Stir the scum back into the liquid before drinking it and you'll notice a marked deterioration in the taste.

It's best not to try storing raw juices, but they can be kept in the fridge for a couple of hours, with a lid on the container. When going on a journey, or forced to spend the day in the alien environment of an office, we do find it beneficial to take along a flask of raw juice to keep us going. Use a large, wide-necked, insulated flask and insert a couple of ice cubes before pouring in your freshly-extracted juice. That way the juice will keep for half a day or longer without losing too much of its wholesomeness. This is definitely a superior refreshment to canned soft drinks.

The Basics

So far, we've talked of fresh fruits and vegetables in more or less the same breath, but before you begin juicing it's important to understand that the two types of juice act within the body in quite different ways. Basically, *fruit* is liquid brain fuel that is particularly useful for detoxifying your body and clearing your mind, while *vegetables* provide the nutritional blocks for rebuilding the metabolic machinery of your body.

Some juice enthusiasts will warn you not to combine fruit and vegetable juices in the same glass, lest they give you wind and cause embarrassing flatulence. In fact this doesn't always happen. The two types of juice can be combined satisfactorily, but in general they don't tend to taste so good together. The exceptions are carrot and apple, which can be mixed with anything.

Carrot is King

During the World War II, propagandists covered up the invention of radar by trying to persuade the enemy that allied fighter pilots were eating so many carrots that they could see in the dark! This hyperbole does, however, contain a grain of truth. Carrots have been repeatedly shown to nourish the optic nerve and significantly improve eyesight in general and night vision in particular. This is but one of the healing properties of the humble carrot, which is the richest source of beta-carotene, the vegetable pigment that gives carrots their glorious orange colour and which the body converts into the cancer-fighting anti-oxidant, vitamin A.

Carrots also contain vitamins C and E, as well as B, D, G and K and the minerals calcium, sodium, potassium, iron and phosphorus. Carrot juice is composed of a combination of elements which nourish the entire system, helping the body to normalise its weight and restore its chemical balance. CJ is incredibly good for you, but recent reports have suggested that eating carrots could be harmful because they contain poisonous pesticide residues.

Not long ago the UK Pesticides Safety Directorate issued a warning after scientists found carrot pesticide residues 25 times higher than they had expected and, in some cases, three times higher than the accepted safety level. The Food Minister was moved to advise the public to remove the tops and peel all carrots, as if that would make them safe. Sadly, the systemic organophosphates concerned don't stop at the skin, they penetrate the whole vegetable. Naturally, therefore, it is always preferable to use organic produce wherever possible.

When it comes to juicing, the carrot is king. It is the most versatile vegetable, with the sweetest juice. If you've only ever tried bottled carrot juice, and didn't like it, don't be put off from trying freshly-extracted CJ, which tastes sublime.

The carotene content of carrots varies considerably and is reflected in the colour. Carrots bought from the supermarket are sometimes almost fluorescent, while organic carrots are a much deeper shade of orange, indicating a much higher concentration of carotene. When buying carrots, choose those with the darkest colour. Although size doesn't really matter, where the recipes in this book refer to a carrot or a number of carrots, as a guide these should be around 15cm (6in) in length.

Whichever variety you use, you'll need about a pound, or half a kilo, of carrots to make 280ml or 10 fl.oz juice. As a rule of thumb, we reckon that half a dozen medium carrots will yield about half a pint of juice. Scrub them under cold running water and remove the tops and tails, but it is not necessary to peel carrots before putting them through the juicer.

Have a Go

Carrot and apple – don't call it Crapple – is the most basic juice cocktail and it tastes so good that, in our experience, nobody has ever turned their nose up at it! Use the *whole* apple except for the woody stem. Apple seeds contain important nourishment too. Start by combining equal parts of the two juices and experiment until you find the proportions that suit you – half and half perhaps, or one part apple to two parts carrot.

Apples are Ace!

If an apple a day keeps the doctor away, a glass or two of freshly-extracted apple juice will keep you regular, boost your immunity to colds, and keep your hair and nails looking lustrous. Apples are full of the soluble dietary fibre, pectin, which makes the juice cloudy, gives it a delightfully creamy texture and acts in the body to clean out toxins and relieve constipation. Apples are also rich in beta-carotene and vitamin C, as well as several B-complex vitamins including B6, and the mineral potassium.

Just as the carrot is the most versatile vegetable when it comes to juicing, apples are the most useful fruit. Apple juice can happily be mixed with any vegetable juice. As such, it is particularly useful in enabling those who are new to juicing slowly to acclimatise themselves to the earthy, wild, raw taste of some freshly extracted juices. Start off by incorporating a lot of apple and gradually reduce the proportion as you become accustomed to the taste and texture of raw juice.

You may be familiar with the taste of juice pressed from various varieties of apple, but you might be surprised by how sweetly smooth and creamy freshly-extracted apple juice is. There are dozens of apple varieties, each with its own distinct flavour, and it's fun to try each one as it appears. In general, you'll find that the greener the apple, the sharper its juice. Golden Delicious are popular, but we find Cox's ideal.

There's no need to peel apples (in fact it's better if you don't) but do wash them thoroughly. Remove the stalk, but not the core. Simply chop them in half and put them through the juicer.

Apples and pears are closely related, but pear trees are less hardy and the fruit more perishable. Pear juice is thick, mild and versatile. It mixes well with other juices, and can be a useful substitute for apple in many recipes. Pears should be washed and the stem removed, then cut to fit your juicer. Mix the juice of two pears with the juice of two apples and drink it down promptly, since this combination oxidises quickly.

Bring on the Berries

Berries are intensely-flavoured vitamin bombs that tend to be high in potassium and contain a remarkable range of other trace elements. Berries have been shown to be particularly good for fighting 'flu and preventing cancer. Strawberries, raspberries, blackberries . . . in fact any berry works well when blended with apple juice, or apple and pear. Juice two apples, one pear and as many berries as you like, or can fit into the glass.

Berries are replete with something called *ellegic acid* – a natural plant *phenol* which is believed to be a powerful anti-cancer/anti-ageing compound. Researchers working with it believe that ellegic acid probably has protective properties because it is taken up by receptor sites that are also used by chemically-induced carcinogens. Animal experiments have demonstrated just how powerful a protective effect ellegic-acid-containing foods have when researchers fed mice on them and then deliberately applied a nasty cancer-causing polycyclic aromatic hydrocarbon (PAH) to the skin for several weeks. The berry-eaters had 45 per cent fewer tumours than the control group and the latency period before they appeared was stretched from six to ten weeks. Berries are also high in potassium and rich in iron. Some, like blackcurrants and redcurrants also contain GLA (a health-giving fatty acid), others like cranberries are great for clearing urinary and bladder infections.

Taking the Pith

When juicing citrus fruit, remove the peel but leave as much of the white pith as you like to get the full benefit of the bioflavonoids contained within it, which help body to absorb vitamin C. Bioflavonoids are powerful plant-based anti-oxidants. They also have an ability to strengthen the capillaries in the body which carry nutrients to the cells via the bloodstream. This means better circulation and smoother, more beautiful skin. The juice of citrus fruits squeezed on a conventional cone juicer often has bits of pith floating in it, which have an unpleasant feel in the mouth. It tends to taste sharp and to cause acidity within the body. Juice that's made using a centrifugal extractor, however, is a whole food in which the citric acid is neutralised by the bioflavonoids, providing the body with a well-balanced drink that can be readily assimilated. It's also absolutely delicious and has a wonderful, creamy texture; it has a sweetness quite unlike squeezed juice.

Citrus juices are jam-packed with fruit sugar and bursting with vitamin C, helping to crank up the immune system and providing instant energy. We find a big glass of frothy pink grapefruit juice just the thing to get us started on a miserable, wet winter morning.

The Whole Juice

The seeds in fruits such as apples and oranges are enormously rich in nutrients. The orange seed has nine times more calcium, seven times more magnesium, and more potassium than an equal amount of orange juice. Apple seeds have five times more potassium than extracted apple juice. Other seeds – those from the rose family such as cherries, peaches, plums, apricots and apples – contain a very small amount of a chemical called amygdalin which is believed to release minute quantities of cyanide. This is not anything that one should be overly concerned about since you would have to consume 50–100 apricot stones to take in a harmful dose. However, we do not suggest you put apricot or cherry stones into the juicer, as they will only blunt the blades.

e incredibly rich in nutrients and they have effect on our health, but it would be quite wrong to describe them as 'concentrated'. As you get into juicing and begin talking to friends about it, you will almost inevitably come across someone who'll try to warn you that too much of a good thing can be bad for you. They might cite the dimly-remembered case of some health fanatic who killed himself with carrot juice. That did actually happen, but the person involved was not only drinking several *gallons* of fresh CJ per day, he was also guzzling toxic doses of vitamin A tablets over months and years to the point where his liver gave up on him. Obviously, he was overdoing it.

When raw juices were first discussed in medical and scientific arenas, it was suggested that they should only be taken in tiny doses, but this was undoubtedly because there wasn't a machine on the market that could easily extract juice in any quantity. Imagine what price you'd put on a glass of carrot juice if you had to grate the vegetable and somehow force it through a super-fine strainer by hand. Now that we have handy centrifugal machines, the recommendation is that you must consume at least a pint of raw juice every day to begin to feel the beneficial effects.

It's true that some juices are very potent and should only be taken in small quantities. However, it will be immediately apparent to you which these juices are because they also have an intensely powerful taste and are too strong to drink straight. Juices are supposed to taste pleasant! The juices of beetroot and broccoli and all leafy, dark green vegetables must be diluted by at least four times the quantity of much milder juices, like carrot and apple, to be palatable.

When you first start juicing, you may well experience some slight discomfort as your body purges itself of toxins and starts to sort itself out, but this is transitory and only to be expected. It's a good idea to start slowly, with no more than a couple of glasses of juice each day. It is virtually impossible to overdose on raw juice – so long, that is, as you don't try to force unnatural quantities of the stuff down yourself. Drink only as much raw juice as feels comfortable. The juices are so delicious you may be tempted to gulp them down. Don't. It is important to drink your juices slowly, sipping them so that all their goodness is absorbed, nothing is wasted and they mix well with salivary enzymes.

The Spice of Life

As you get into juicing and become accustomed to the staple combinations, you will soon lose any inhibitions you may have nurtured about tasting more pungent and increasingly earthy juices. It's important that you do. Carrot & Apple, or Carrot & Orange juices are all very well, in fact they're terrific. But to derive the maximum benefit from your juicer, it's vital that you consume as broad a variety of fruits and vegetables as possible. Leafy green vegetables are particularly important for good health, as we'll see in Chapter Seven, but they can taste foul at first. The trick is to gradually incorporate more green – more cabbage, spinach, dandelion, etc – into your juices as you become accustomed to the taste.

Raw juices can be spiced up with the addition of root ginger, or fresh garlic, but easy does it. Both have strong flavours, which can be overpowering, and garlic in particular can have an overwhelming effect. Don't use more than one clove per glass of juice and wash the juicer out thoroughly immediately after using garlic, for it is likely to become contaminated and to continue flavouring your juices for days to come. Ginger need not be peeled, just cut into cubes of about a centimetre.

However you choose to get into juicing, the important thing is simply to get started and see where it takes you. Juice-making is a highly creative sport. There is always some delicious new combination just waiting to be discovered.

Chapter Three
Juice Blitz

'Detox' has become a buzz-word of the late 20th century, but it is not a recent fad. For thousands of years, detoxification rituals have been used by mystics and shamen in order to attain a state of heightened spirituality. Ritual fasting, with the conviction that abstinence brings us closer to God, is a feature of many religions. On a secular level, many Westerners periodically spend time at health farms in order to give their battered bodies a break from rich food, poor air and the stresses and strains of modern life.

Detoxification is the process of eliminating stored wastes from the body and is the first step in curing addiction. If you are determined to give up cigarettes, for example, the Juice Blitz will help you. By consuming nothing but raw juice and spring water for 36 hours, not only will you remove the temptation to smoke after meals or over a drink, but you will facilitate the process of elimination and help to flush the nicotine out of your body. In fact, the Juice Blitz can be a useful tool in the withdrawal stage of treatment for any form of substance abuse. Then, of course, the addict has to alter the behavioural patterns that reinforce his or her addiction.

Juice High

If you have never, ever, over-indulged in any processed or chemically-treated or preserved food, if you've never smoked a cigarette, done drugs or got drunk, then you probably don't need to detox your body. But how many of us have led that kind of blameless and boring life? Bearing in mind all the junk you've put into your body over the years, you'll realise that you can't get rid of it all overnight. Like housework, the Juice Blitz takes a little effort, but the end result more than makes it all worth-while. It's not easy to change the eating habits of a life-time, but the Juice Blitz will enable you to make a fresh start.

Juice Freedom

Remember that there is nothing in raw juice that your body can't use. By going for 36 hours without consum-ing anything but raw juice, you will be giving your body a break and relieving it of the hard work of digestion. Left to its own devices, the body will automatically initiate a wholesale house-cleaning. A small minority of people find this process uncomfortable. If you experience any of the reactions described in the 'Trouble Shooting' table (see pages 44–45), take it as an indication that this cleansing process is well under way and that your body is purging itself. And be glad for that.

You may be pleasantly surprised by the effect that blitz-ing your body has on your mind. Many people experience an amazing mind lift almost as soon as they stop clogging their bodies with junk and start flushing their system. Considering the synergistic relationship of the body and mind, it should be obvious that lightening the body's workload will free the mind to roam fresh horizons.

Fasting on raw juices is probably the most potent short-term antidote to stress. What's more, we find that if we have a lot of work to do that requires our full concentration over long periods, it's also a great way to meet deadlines! Whenever we feel run-down and jaded, or in need of a clearer head, the Juice Blitz can not only reinvigorate our bodies, but also clear mental blockages, and help us to get a better perspective on difficult problems or vexatious situations. Sometimes, we find ourselves living on nothing but raw juice for a day or two at a stretch just because it feels so good.

Crash Detox

The Juice Blitz is a crash course designed to introduce novices to the state of being Juice High. It can be performed at home over the weekend since this will probably give you a chance for more rest. From, say, Friday night to Sunday lunchtime, all you will be putting into your body is freshly-extracted raw juice. If this sounds arduous, then be reassured that you won't go hungry. Although it doesn't sit heavily in your stomach, raw juice completely satisfies the appetite. Most people find themselves perfectly happy with four to six glasses over the course of the day. However, you can drink more than that so long as you don't overdo it. Have spring water too, if you like. Let your body be the judge of how much you need.

The eight juice recipes given below demonstrate some of the classic juice combinations that you might use after, as well as during, your Juice Blitz. They promote effective elimination and provide all the raw energy your body needs for the valuable work of deep cleansing. They are listed in the order that they should be consumed during the day, with the fruit juices to be drunk in the morning and the more savoury, earthier vegetable cocktails to be taken as the day wears on. You're not required to make use of all these recipes, or even to stick to them. The recipes are highly adaptable (for more variations see Recipes, p.112) and the possible combinations of raw juice are infinite, so feel free to improvise. But don't abandon the principle of drinking fruit juices *before* vegetable juices. Here is what the Blitz regime looks like:

THE NIGHT BEFORE

Start your Juice Blitz by going to bed a little hungry the night before. For dinner, drink a glass of the More Raw NRG cocktail or Potassium Punch (see pages 38 and 39). These are ideal, because their exceptional potassium content will counteract the acidity in your body and set up the optimum conditions for your body to do its work. Unless diluted with spring water, the root vegetable drinks may seem a little heavy for beginners to handle at this early stage in the game.

JUICE BLITZ DAY

Start the next morning with a melon or citrus juice and continue with fruit juices until midday. For lunch, try one of the more potent vegetable cocktails, like the Beet Treat (see page 40), which is a great source of sustained energy to carry you through the day. Throughout the afternoon and early evening, stick to vegetable juices in which apple is the only fruit ingredient. We find the More Raw NRG cocktail (see page 38) to be the most useful while detoxing, adding dark green leaves of spinach or watercress or even dandelion to increase its vitality.

Over the course of the first day of a juice fast, you may experience the odd sensation that is not entirely pleasurable. You might find yourself suddenly irritable, or tired, or you could even develop a mild headache. The best antidote to any of these symptoms is to lie down in a darkened room and take a nap. If you have been able to give over your weekend to the Juice Blitz, rest as much as possible and let your body do its work in peace. In any case, rest as much as possible. Don't attempt any strenuous exercise while you are blitzing, but a gentle stroll in fresh air is always a good idea.

BLITZ NIGHT & MORNING AFTER

On Blitz night avoid consuming anything except water after 8 o'clock. You might like to take a long, languorous bath. If you can find a friend to share it with and scrub your back, so much the better. Perhaps your friend can be persuaded to give you a massage as well. The best thing to do on Saturday night while you're blitzing is to go to bed early and get a good night's sleep. If you're not sleepy, go to bed anyway. If you're going to bed alone, take a juicy novel or a lurid video to keep yourself entertained.

The morning after, start the day once again with fruit juice. After a good night's rest, you are likely to be feeling full of the joys of life. Even if your night was not particularly restful and you found yourself waking at dawn in a pool of sweat, you will probably feel sharper, mentally. If you customarily do a crossword in the Sunday papers, we bet you'll find that you finish it faster than usual. You may also find sudden surges of energy, accompanied by some mental agitation. These are both symptoms that your metabolism has been cranked into high gear and the best antidote is a brisk walk in fresh air.

RAW ENERGY LUNCH

As you approach lunchtime on the second day and the end of your Juice Blitz, you may be faced with the predicament of having to sit down to a large, traditional meal or risk offending your mum, or the person who cooked it. You might even be looking forward to stuffing yourself. Don't. Your first meal should be composed of at least 75 per cent raw foods. That means plenty of salad . . .

Ease yourself back into the routine of normal meals by eating smaller portions and by taking care to chew every mouthful thoroughly. That way you will be better able to appreciate the taste of your food and it will be digested more quickly.

THE REST OF YOUR LIFE

Should you wish to carry on blitzing and to continue your juice fast through two whole days, fine. The longer you maintain your Juice Blitz, the more deep-cleansing your body can accomplish at a cellular level. But don't overdo it. Your body can't reverse the negative effects of years on a poor diet in a single week, or even a month. The Juice Blitz is intended to jump-start a process that it may take years to complete. It is not a way of life. You'll know how long you can maintain a juice fast because your body will tell you when it's over by making you overwhelmingly hungry!

As soon as you experience extreme pangs of hunger, break your fast. If, at any time while blitzing, you experience symptoms more serious than those listed under 'Trouble Shooting' (pages 44–45), consult your doctor or medical advisor. If you are contemplating a juice fast lasting longer than two or three days, it's a good idea to consult a health practitioner who is experienced in juice therapy before you begin.

The Plan

Before you start blitzing, do a little forward planning. You are going to need a fair quantity of fruits and vegetables, so make a list before you shop to ensure you remember everything. Where possible, always buy fruits and vegetables that have been grown organically, without the use of chemical fertilisers and pesticides. Often, organic produce doesn't look as good as the cheaper stuff that's displayed in the supermarket, but it is inherently better for you because none of its nutritional integrity has been compromised. People are waking up to the truth of this statement so rapidly that there is a shortage of organic produce across Europe and it might not be easy for you to locate a supplier, but it is quite definitely worth the effort.

Over the course of the weekend, your biggest enemy may well be boredom. Breaking from your usual dietary regime is never completely effortless and if you are bored you might well suffer hunger pangs and be tempted to start snacking. So find something to preoccupy your mind over the weekend. Read novels or watch videos; write letters or telephone friends you haven't seen for a while.

BLITZ ESSENTIALS: THE EIGHT GREAT ELIMINATORS

Merry Belon

Melons go through the system faster than any other fruit and are therefore recommended by many juice experts to be drunk on their own. The key to the melon's efficacy is the exceptionally high water content of the flesh, while the nutrients are concentrated in the rind and skin, which can and should also be juiced. Some melons like honeydew and cantaloupes have waxy or netted skins which can be trimmed off with a decent vegetable peeler. Others, like watermelons, can be simply scrubbed, sliced to fit your juicer and put through the machine, seeds and all.

Melons in general and watermelons in particular are a perfect source of the fluids your body needs on a daily basis and a good source of B-complex vitamins, as well as being rich in vitamin C. There is an ever-growing profusion of melon varieties on the market, and it's fun to experiment with all of them. But melon juice can be a bit on the bland side. The addition of a handful of succulent summer berries will brighten it up considerably.

Berries are the one fruit that combines really well with melons and the array of flavours gives lots of scope for experimentation. In hot weather, a good tip is to freeze your berries before juicing them. Try Galia & Raspberry, Honeydew & Blackberry or the classic Watermelon & Strawberry:

1 slice of watermelon, 3cm wide and cut into chunks to fit your juicer

6 strawberries, washed and with their green stalks removed

Citrus Zinger

Whole citrus juice freshly-extracted using a centrifugal machine has a homogenised, creamy texture and tastes like sherbet. The pith of grapefruit is especially rich in bioflavonoids, which is hardly surprising since grapefruit juice tends to be the most bitter of the citrus family. Pink grapefruits are sweeter and juicier than plain yellow ones and you have to pay a premium price for them, but it's worth it. It's sometimes hard to get hold of good, juicy oranges but the Mandarin varieties, like tangerines, are a good substitute in the depths of winter.

The skin of citrus fruits is often waxed to preserve its shelf life and, therefore, should always be removed. Even a sliver of lemon peel put through your juicer can ruin the taste of your juice. Use lemons and limes sparingly, never adding more than half of either fruit to a glass of juice. The following recipe is a mélange of citrus spiked with ginger for an intriguing aftertaste. Feel free to vary it as you like:

1 orange	*1/2 lemon or lime*
1 pink grapefruit	*1cm cube of ginger (optional)*

Fab 5 Fruit Juice

You can vary the fruit content as you like and depending on what you are able to buy, you can substitute a clementine or satsuma for the tangerine, white grapes for red, and pineapple or mango for the peach. Apples and pears should be cut to fit your juicer and put through the machine, pips and all. Remove the stones from peaches and mangoes. Cut the fibrous skin from pineapples and slice them into long spears. This fruit mix is thick and frothy with a pleasant, balanced flavour that's especially good on a warm day when you might like to add some ice cubes to it and sip it slowly through a straw:

1/2 apple	*A dozen red grapes*
1/2 pear	*1 peach*
1 tangerine	

Sweet Salvation

Sweet capsicums (peppers) produce a juice with amazing colour and fantastic flavour, but they also contain more vitamin C than oranges. Sadly, many peppers these days are grown for looks rather than flavour. Pick the ones with the deepest colour and wash them well before use. Freshly-made tomato juice bears little relation to the canned variety and reminds us of why these succulent, savoury fruit were once called love apples. Look for vine-ripened tomatoes, which have better flavour. This cocktail has a deep red-orange colour and can be a bit thick. Dilute it with the judicious addition of cucumber, which should be peeled before it is juiced unless it is organically grown.

1 red or yellow pepper
2 ripe tomatoes (or 1 beef tomato)

1–2 carrots
3cm section of cucumber

More Raw NRG

Like the plain Raw NRG cocktail in Recipes (p.124), More Raw is based on the crucial combination of carrot and apple, with green vegetable juices diluted by cucumber and celery. The juice extracted from green veggies is very powerful, both in its healthful properties and its taste. Spinach and watercress are invaluable for conditioning the entire digestive system thanks to the oxalic acid they contain, which helps to maintain the action of peristalsis. They are also amongst the best sources of vitamins C and E. Dandelion leaves are the first spring greens to sprout. They're an excellent source of calcium and potassium and the best known source of beta-carotene among the green vegetables. No wonder rabbits love them.

You will find the green juices a little strong at first, and will need to dilute them with cucumber and celery, but as you get used to the taste you can incorporate more leaves into your juices. When making this juice, put the ingredients through your juicer in this order and you'll end up with a greenish drink tinged with orange froth:

1 small bunch of spinach or
   watercress (or dandelion)
   leaves
1 floret of broccoli

3cm section of cucumber
2 stalks of celery
1 apple
3 carrots

Potassium Punch

This recipe is our tribute to N.W. Walker, the American raw food pioneer and proponent of natural healing who helped to develop the technique of juicing and was one of the first to write about the wonders of raw juice. A marvellous testament to the truth of the idea that you are what you eat, Dr Walker lived to the age of 106. An evangelist of detoxification, he would recommend to his patients that they drink his Raw Potassium Broth, although he would be the first to admit that most people don't find it as palatable as straight carrot juice or concoctions based on a carrot and apple mix.

In the words of the great man himself: 'The organic minerals and salts in this combination of raw potassium 'broth' embrace practically the entire range of those required by the body. Its effect in reducing excessive acidity in the stomach has been truly remarkable. There is probably no food more complete in every respect than this for the human organism.' So there you have it. We recommend that you drink at least a glass a day.

3 carrots
2 stalks celery
4–6 leaves of lettuce or winter
   greens
A handful of spinach or
   watercress (or dandelion)
   leaves

A few stalks of fresh coriander or
   parsley

Beet Treat

You have to be careful how you handle beetroot juice, which is most valuable for flushing the kidneys and enriching the blood, but can cause a dramatic cleansing action if taken in quantities of more than half a glass at a time. Cut the fibrous root off the bottom of your beets, but there's no need to peel them so long as they're thoroughly washed. You can include the leafy tops, too, if they are attached. The juice has a wonderful purple colour and an earthy, wholesome flavour. But don't overdo it. Take it from us that too much beet juice is liable to provoke a profoundly moving experience!

½ whole beetroot, including the
leafy top if possible
2 carrots

1 apple
1 stalk of celery
3cm section of cucumber

Roots Soup

Root vegetables are the best source of thiamin, riboflavin, niacin and other water-soluble vitamins of the B complex and are abundant in trace elements. Their juices are thick, sweet and creamy and are complemented by the slightly aniseed flavour of fennel, which adds an intriguing dimension to this recipe. Fennel is a folk cure for heartburn in the Cajun country of Louisiana and a darned effective one at that. Dilute your root soup with cucumber juice, but if it's still too thick add a splash of spring water.

½ beetroot
1 medium-sized parsnip
1 sweet potato

½ bulb of fennel
5cm section of cucumber

Breathing & Brushing

The Juice Blitz will accelerate the detoxification of your body from within by flushing the bowels and kidneys, but these are only two of the routes by which toxins are expelled. Just as important are the lungs and the skin. While detoxing, it's important to pay special attention to both.

Breathing is the most fundamental process of life. It goes without saying that if you were deprived of oxygen, you'd expire within minutes, but no less crucial is the second half of the respiratory process: discarding carbon dioxide by breathing out. CO_2 is the poisonous by-product of oxidation and energy release in your cells which is carried back to the lungs in the blood and eliminated when you breathe out. At least that's how it *should* work but, since most of us use less than half of our breathing capacity, the system rarely functions as efficiently as it might. Learning to breathe properly is an elementary step towards reconditioning your body.

Most of us breathe with only the top half of our bodies, but proper breathing requires the use of the diaphragm, the muscle that separates the chest cavity from the abdomen. When you breathe correctly, the diaphragm contracts, allowing the lungs to expand and fill with air. During a single day, the average person will breathe in more than 11,000 litres of air. To make the best use of it all you must learn to breathe deeply, from the bottom up. You can ensure proper breathing and keep your lungs working well by taking a daily dose of aerobic exercise. In addition the following deep breathing exercise will be a great help:

1. Go outside into the fresh air, or open a window.
2. Stand with your feet slightly apart and your hands on your sides, touching your lower ribs just above the waist.
3. Inhale through your nose for the slow count of five and feel how your abdomen swells as you do so.
4. Continue to breathe in for another count of five, filling your lungs and expanding your rib cage.
5. Hold your breath for another count of five.
6. Exhale slowly through the mouth for the count of ten, noticing how your ribcage shrinks as you do so and pulling in with your abdominal muscles until you have expelled all the air.
7. Repeat this exercise four times.

Not only does breathing enable us to take in oxygen and expel CO_2, it also keeps the lymphatic system moving. These lymphatics are the body's sewage system: an elaborate network of microscopic channels that covers the whole body and is filled with a clear liquid called lymph. This is the medium by which nutrients are carried into the tissues of your body and metabolic waste is removed. There's more lymph in your body than blood and the lymphatic system is similar to the tiny capillaries of the pulmonary system, but with one vital difference. Whereas blood is pumped around your body by your heart, lymph has no pump and is only kept flowing by gravity and by muscular movement.

Get Moving

One of the best techniques for encouraging lymphatic drainage and spring-cleaning your body is known as skin brushing. It stimulates the movement of interstitial fluids and breaks down congestion in areas where the flow of lymph has become sluggish. Gentle yet powerful, it takes only five minutes in the morning or evening before your bath or shower and is both invigorating and pleasurable:

1. Use a natural-fibre brush with quite a long handle, or a loofah.
2. Begin at the tips of your shoulders and cover your whole body (except the head), working downwards, with long, smooth strokes over the shoulders, arms and trunk.
3. Starting at the feet, brush upwards over the legs and hips.

You need only go over your skin once for the brushing to be effective. Regular brushing will stimulate lymph-flow and unclog the pores of your skin. How firmly you press depends entirely on how well-toned your skin is. Go easy to begin with and become more vigorous as your skin gets fitter.

JUICE BLITZ: QUICK REFERENCE

The Night Before	Juice Blitz Day	Blitz Night & Morning After	The Rest of Your Life
For dinner, a glass of the More Raw NRG cocktail or Potassium Punch	Start with a melon or citrus juice and continue with fruit juices all day. Lunch: try a Beet Treat. Stick to vegetable juices (mixed with apple if desired) throughout the day.	Drink nothing but water after 8 o'clock. Start the next morning with fruit juice. Lunch: plenty of salad – your first meal after the Blitz should be 75 per cent raw foods.	The longer you maintain the Juice Blitz the more deep-cleansing your body will do. But don't overdo it. Break your fast as soon as you experience extreme pangs of hunger. The Juice Blitz is a jump-start for a process that may take years to complete. It is not a way of life but an invaluable tool.

TROUBLE SHOOTING

Most people experience no discomfort while blitzing their bodies with juice, but there are always exceptions. A small percentage of people, those whose systems are particularly toxic (and therefore most in need of detoxification) may experience one or more of the symptoms listed below. If this applies to you, don't let yourself be discouraged from continuing with the Juice Blitz for the full 36 hours. Remember that these complaints are not the signs of illness developing in your body, but of the toxins that cause illness leaving it. Recognise that they are temporary and will leave you feeling better than ever.

Bloating and/or Flatulence	This is quite common at the start of the Juice Blitz when you start consuming freshly-extracted fruit juices on an empty stomach. Its cleansing action will sluice the walls of your stomach and stir up accumulated food debris, causing wind. Look on it as the body girding itself for the work ahead.
Diarrhoea	What you may think of as diarrhoea probably isn't and certainly should not be anything to worry about. Raw juice will wash impacted faeces from your intestinal walls and expel it from the bowel in the form of loose, runny stools. This is highly beneficial and will leave you feeling lighter and renewed.

Headaches, Mood Swings, Irritability	These are all symptomatic of the chemical change in your body and are easily overcome if you understand them as a sign that the detoxification is starting to have its effect. Take a nap, go for a walk, or do the deep breathing exercise described above.
Tiredness and Boredom	The hard work of detoxifying your body requires a lot of energy, so it's quite natural to feel sleepy. Being bored is the result of inadequate preparation. Surely you can find something to amuse yourself with? Read, watch videos, play games. Just stay out of the pub.
Catarrh	Caught a cold? Actually, a copious discharge of mucus from your nasal passage rarely indicates a viral infection but is one of the classic ways in which the body eliminates stored toxins. So blow your snotty nose and be glad you're getting rid of them.
Perspiration	Your skin is the largest organ of elimination and the most direct route out of your body for a lot of toxins. Consequently, if you find that you perspire more heavily than usual while blitzing, particularly while you're asleep in bed, don't worry about it. If you are using the Juice Blitz to stop smoking, you are liable to lose quite a lot of fluid as your body takes the opportunity to expel the nicotine through the pores of the skin.

Chapter Four
Body Building

Juice drinking works two kinds of magic on your body. The first is detoxification. Detox is central not only to healing illness but to protecting from degeneration as well as to regenerating and rejuvenating the body. That is why it forms the basis of every form of natural medicine in the world. The principle is simple: clean out the body and you raise vitality, strengthen its healing powers and set it free from the burden of chronic fatigue and heaviness that plagues the majority of men and women in industrialized countries these days. Once, detox itself was probably enough to heal and boost vitality. Now, as a result of widespread nutritional deficiencies, it is only half of what is called for. Now we need to look not only at how to *detox* the system but how to *rebuild* its metabolic pathways. We call this process body building.

Get a Life

As a result of the way we have depleted our foods of essential nutrients and distorted the vitamin and mineral balance in our bodies through chemical farming, heavy food processing, and long storage of our foods, most of us have nowhere near the optimal levels of vitamins, minerals and vital trace elements our bodies need to be superhealthy. Many nutrients – from vitamin B6 to the mineral zinc and the trace element silicon – must be present both in adequate amounts and in a good balance in order to stimulate the activity of enzymes on which every life process depends.

Your body cannot make its own minerals. It has to take them in, in a good balance, from the foods you eat.

In addition to nitrogen, potassium and phosphorus, the body requires magnesium, manganese and calcium, selenium, zinc, copper, iodine, boron, molybdenum, vanadium and probably other elements as yet undiscovered.

Organic Magic

The organic matter in healthy soil is Nature's factory for biological activity. It is built up as a result of the breakdown of vegetable and animal matter by the soil's natural 'residents' – worms, bacteria and other useful micro-organisms. The presence of these creatures in the right quantity and type gives rise to physical, chemical and biological properties that create fertility in our soils and make plants grown on them highly resistant to disease. When it comes to human health they do a lot more. The minerals and trace elements we need to trigger the metabolic processes *must* be in an organic form. That is, they need to be taken from living things like plant or animal foods. You cannot eat nails – inorganic iron – and expect to protect yourself from anaemia, or chew sand – inorganic silica – and be sure to get enough of the trace element to keep your nails and hair strong and help protect your bones from osteoporosis. It is the organic matter in soils that enables plants grown on them to transform inorganic iron and silica into the organic form which is taken up by the vegetables and fruits, grains and legumes grown on them. Organic methods of farming help protect against significant distortions in mineral balances – that is from an increase in one or more mineral elements which can alter the availability of others and undermine health. No such protection is available when foods are chemically grown.

Making Do

The deficiencies we are developing through eating chemically grown and processed foods have brought metabolic distortions in their wake – such as degenerative diseases, early ageing, and emotional disturbances like depression and anxiety. These kinds of deficiencies cannot easily be corrected. Popping the latest multi-mineral tablet from your corner pharmacy or health-food store won't do it. Daily juicing will.

Nutrients in foods exist in complex synergy and affect each other. They interact and work together in your body. The balance of bio-available minerals and trace elements needed in the body for peak well-being is infinitely more complex than vitamin fanatics would have us believe. This is where raw juices really come into their own. To restore biochemical balance once it has been disturbed, you need a continual supply of the vitamins and minerals as well as other health-enhancing substances that are found in fresh vegetables and fruits and in green plants such as seaweeds, spirulina, chlorella, barley grass or alfalfa.

Perfect Synergy

Recent research has focused on seeking out and identifying specific nutrients and compounds – called phyto-chemicals – that are present within common foods and that appear to act naturally to prevent cancer and other diseases. Thanks to the particular balance of amino acids, enzymes, polysaccharides and other compounds they contain, such foods as garlic, licorice, and green compounds like green barley, spirulina, chlorella and many other fresh foods have the ability to turn on the human immune system. Some contain *isoflavones* and *protease inhibitors* (see p.50) which are capable of breaking down layers surrounding foreign proteins, including tumours. Others are rich in *phyto-sterols* (see p.49), useful in protecting both men and women from reproductive damage by herbicides and pesticides (which act as oestrogen-mimics or *xenoestrogens* to lower sperm count in men and encourage PMS, osteoporosis, endometriosis and fibroids in women).

Blinkered Nutrition

One of the problems with most of the information that is handed out through the media and books on nutrition is that it is highly fragmented. You hear talk about a specific vitamin or mineral and how we should take more of it, about cholesterol or protein or fibre. We seem to have become obsessed in recent years with breaking everything down and looking at the effects of specific ingredients on our bodies. We have forgotten how to see the wood for the trees. It is not just the ingredient – a particular vitamin or mineral or compound – in a vegetable that can do us good. It is the synergy of nature, in which the whole is far greater than the sum of its parts.

Protective Compounds

In fresh fruits and vegetables, phyto-chemicals come in a total package. Here are some of the most important of the specific ingredients so far identified:

saponins: these have anti-oxidant properties and as such help prevent changes to the cells' DNA (our genetic coding) associated with premature ageing and the development of cancer. Research shows that cancer of the colon is much lower in populations where there is a high dietary intake of saponins.

phyto-sterols: these plant hormones include such chemicals as *stigmasterol* and *ergosterol* which are little absorbed in the digestive system. They pass on to the colon where they help prevent damage from the cancer-producing breakdown products from cholesterol. Some phyto-sterols are also weak oestrogenic compounds capable of binding with oestrogen receptor sites in both male and female bodies, protecting against reproductive problems that develop as a result of exposure to xenoestrogens. Many phyto-sterols also help protect against premature ageing of the skin and skin cancer as well as prostate troubles, PMS and menopausal miseries.

phenolic acids: these anti-oxidants help prevent damage to cellular DNA associated with premature ageing and the development of degenerative diseases.

protease inhibitors: these compounds help protect against the damaging effects of toxins in the body and against radiation and free radical damage. In laboratory studies protease inhibitors have been shown to inhibit cancers of the mouth, pancreas, lung, colon and digestive tract. Unfortunately protease inhibitors – which exist in good quantities in many common wholesome foods including potatoes, eggs, and grains – are greatly destroyed by cooking. In many raw vegetables, however, they are in rich supply.

omega-3 fatty acids: these are essential fatty acids which, when unadulterated by heating or processing and taken fresh, have been shown to protect against cancer and heart disease. They also play important roles in the manufacture of hormones in the body and are found in good quantities in flaxseeds or linseeds, in sprouted seeds and grains which you can use for juicing, and in some of the special green foods such as spirulina.

isoflavones: these are plant hormones which carry strong anti-cancer properties, particularly in relation to cancers of the reproductive system such as prostate cancer, cervical cancer, ovarian cancer, endometrial cancer and breast cancer. The molecular structure of isoflavonoids is very close to that of the oestrogens, but they are only one hundred-thousandth as potent as the body's oestrogens and oestrogens given in the form of drugs. Eating foods or making juices of foods rich in the isoflavones can help protect both men and women from xenoestrogens in the environment. Japanese researchers have shown that the weak oestrogenic effect of isoflavones can relieve – often even completely eliminate – the negative symptoms associated with PMS and menopause.

Plant compounds play an important, if not yet fully understood, part in restoring the kind of biochemical balance that the body's metabolic processes need to function smoothly. You need only examine a couple of common vegetables to see just how powerful the protective, restoring plant compounds they contain can be.

Caring Carrot

Carrots are unbelievably rich in anti-oxidant and cancer-preventive compounds. The most well known of these is beta-carotene. This naturally occurring anti-oxidant has become famous in recent years as a safe-to-take precursor to vitamin A – something that your body can turn into vitamin A as needed. But beta-carotene is only the most well-researched of the carotinoids. Scientists are now discovering many others which appear to have equal if not greater health-supporting abilities. A high consumption of foods containing carotinoids has been shown to lower the incidence of lung, pancreas and prostate cancer. Even cancer among cigarette smokers is lower among people with carotinoid-rich diets. So much is this true that smokers on carotinoid-poor diets are four times more likely to get cancer than those who consume the carotinoids in even one carrot a day. Think how much more you get when you drink a full glass of fresh carrot juice each day. Carotinoids are by no means the only goodies in carrot juice, nor are carrots the only place that you will find good quantities of them. Spirulina – which is a wonderful green additive to juices – is ultra-rich in carotinoids, as are winter marrow, yams and other green vegetables.

Carrots also contain other fabulous health-boosting friends such as MOP – a little compound with an amazing ability to help repair DNA. Damage to DNA is the central cause of degeneration and premature ageing in the body. Prevent it and you can prevent early ageing. That is where MOP comes in. MOP actually tucks itself in between the base pairs of DNA molecules and repairs damage that has occurred. Scientists experimenting with MOP have found that they can take damaged white blood cells from people, add MOP to them and then put the white blood cells back into the body in perfect shape. Parsnips are also rich in MOP and mix well with carrot juice.

Green Glory

There are an amazing thirty-three cancer-preventive compounds in fresh broccoli. These include beta-carotene and indole-3-carbinol which have the ability to counteract many of the chemicals which pollute our environment – such as the *nitrosamines* which are known to cause cancer. (Nitrosamines are formed when nitrites are used to preserve and colour meat.) Indole-3-carbinol not only prevents cancer but also helps prevent other degenerative diseases as well as premature ageing. A cup full of broccoli or one of the other dark greens in a glass of carrot and apple juice once a day delivers 165 per cent of the recommended daily allowance for vitamin C, 40 per cent for vitamin A and 20 per cent for calcium.

Natural Healing

Most people have never heard of the indoles or saponins or any of the other fresh food compounds that can encourage radiant health – although volumes have been written about their virtues in scientific literature. Even more esoteric is the knowledge about how juices made from fresh raw foods enhance health not from a *chemical* point of view but rather from an *energetic* one. World experts in natural healing have made remarkable use of raw foods and their juices to help the body eliminate cancer from its system, cure migraine, rejuvenate, and improve athletic performance.

Back to Basics

Human evolution is a slow process. For hundreds of generations our ancestors lived on wild foods gathered and eaten raw. Our genes appear to be specially adapted to dealing with raw foods. The famous Swiss physician Max Bircher-Benner and the German Max Gerson used living foods not only to support the human organism's healing but also to heighten vitality as well as to regenerate and rejuvenate the body as a whole. By incorporating a good percentage of live foods – fresh vegetables, raw seeds and nuts, fresh sprouted grains and seeds and especially fresh vegetable juices – in your diet you can help rebalance hormones, stabilize moods, clear and rejuvenate skin, shed excess fat stores and transform your emotional and spiritual outlook on life.

More than fifty years ago the distinguished Viennese doctor Hans Eppinger discovered that a high-raw way of eating leads to increased cellular respiration. It does this in a number of ways, creating a kind of positive feedback loop which leads to heightened cell metabolism. It eliminates accumulated wastes and toxins from cells and tissues. It supplies the level of nutrients essential for optimal cell function. And, perhaps most important of all, it heightens the micro-electrical tensions associated with cell vitality so that even cells in a particularly sluggish and neglected system are revitalized. They become better able to burn calories in the presence of oxygen and to produce energy efficiently both for overall vitality and for carrying out the housekeeping on which the health of your body depends.

Micro-Electrics

Capillaries are minute blood vessels which form a vast network of microcirculation throughout your body. It is their responsibility to deliver oxygen-rich blood for it to be used by the cells. So important are these fine vessels that nature has supplied you with incredible lengths of them. If you were to attach all the capillaries in your body end to end they would measure some 60,000 miles in length – more than twice around the world. The condition of your body as a whole depends to a great extent on the state of your capillaries. As the arbitrators of cell nutrition, respiration and elimination, capillaries carry nutrients and oxygen around your body. Each of them has tiny 'pores' which allow plasma (but not red blood cells) to seep through and pass into the body fluid. This is how nutrients are delivered and wastes eliminated from tissues. Without good microcirculation, metabolism cannot take place efficiently. That is why the capillaries play a vital part in the successful elimination of excess fat deposits with all their stored toxins.

Unfortunately, over the years the capillaries of people living on the average western diet (with its excessive fats, proteins and refined and processed food) become twisted, distended and highly porous. When this happens, proteins seep through and deposit themselves between the tissues and the capillary walls, where they interfere with proper oxygen exchange and impede nutrient delivery and waste elimination. This can gradually starve cells, tissues and organs of all they need to function properly and can also lower cellular metabolic activity. In this deprived condition the entire organism (i.e. your body) is predisposed to degenerative illness and to rapid ageing. A Juice High lifestyle, drinking three or four glasses of freshly made juice, at least two of which are primarily vegetable juices, helps restore normal microcirculation. This in turn heightens metabolism, keeping your weight down and maintaining a high level of energy.

Dynamic Tensions

The interchange of chemicals and energy between the microcirculation and the cells takes place through two thin membranes and a fine interstitial space. And it happens only because the cells and capillaries have what is known as 'selective capacity'. This means they are able to absorb the substances they need and to reject what is harmful or unnecessary for metabolic processes. This selective capacity is the result of antagonistic chemical and micro-electrical tensions in the cells and tissues of all living systems. When you suffer from a chronic degenerative condition or when metabolism is lowered these micro-electrical tensions are drastically reduced. The stronger the tensions – the more intense these antagonisms – the healthier and more vital your body will be and the more efficiently it will be able to burn off stored fat and eliminate toxicity. The chronic fatigue and lowered metabolism which typically occur in women as they grow older – particularly if they have been on and off low-calorie slimming regimes over the years – is accompanied by a decrease in chemical and micro-electrical tensions and a loss of selective capacity. Cell reproduction slows down, capillary walls are weakened and there is a gradual build-up in the interstitial spaces of a sticky 'marsh' derived from excess waste products. This marsh, or tissue sludge, impedes biochemical processes including the production and balancing of hormones and tends to lower metabolism even further, impairing the efficient elimination of wastes by the lymph system.

The lymph nodes, which are located in the groin and under the arm and the neck, filter the lymphatic fluid to remove impurities and dead cells; they are also a place where antibodies, which fight infection or toxins, are made. After purification at the nodes, the fluid is returned to the blood. However, when the lymph system becomes clogged or does not eliminate properly the body can become seriously burdened with toxicity.

Excess toxicity is the common factor in the development of degenerative diseases such as arthritis, cancer, heart disease and diabetes as well as early ageing, the development of persistent cellulite in women's bodies and the tendency to store and to maintain a high level of fat deposits in both men and women.

Increase Selective Capacity

Eppinger and another German scientist, Karl Eimer, showed why drinking live juices and eating lots of fresh raw vegetables can change all this. They steadily *increase* selective capacity by heightening electrical potentials between tissue cells and capillary blood. This improves the ability of your capillaries to regulate the transport of nutrients. It also helps detoxify the system, removing any sticky marsh of waste products that may be present. A way of eating that is high in living foods and their juices, where say 50 per cent of what you eat is taken raw, together with regular exercise, breaks through that vicious circle of fatigue replacing it with a well-functioning metabolism which makes detoxification and the rebuilding of the body's metabolism a steady, straightforward occurrence.

Drink lots of raw juices and choose the rest of your foods from wholesome natural products such as grains and pulses, sea plants, fresh vegetables, fresh locally-grown fruits, and tofu, and you will notice a dramatic improvement in how you look and feel and function within the first couple of weeks. But it will be several weeks before the burden of toxicity which you have been carrying has fully cleared, and it will probably be a few months before even deeper benefits begin to show themselves. By then any pre-existing subclinical vitamin or mineral deficiencies should clear up completely. So be patient. Your body has a quite magnificent ability to heal itself and to excel at being superhealthy, but this doesn't happen overnight.

Chapter Five
High Life

The Juice Blitz is a first-rate, quick-fix detox regime that gives you an intimation of the Juice High lifestyle. Once you've experienced its clear-headed benefits, you'll want to take it further. The next step, as we've just seen, is *body building*, using raw juices to replenish lost vitamins, mineral and trace elements, and to help prevent degenerative diseases as well as energise, regenerate and rejuvenate your body. The High Life Diet will give you all the support you need to carry on the good work.

High Life is an exciting, delicious food style for the future which satisfies the senses and fuels the body so that it functions at peak efficiency on an on-going basis. Its high raw food content and its dependence on wholesome *real* food – instead of the ersatz packaged stuff that these days masquerades as food – provides the kind of high quality nutrition you require to feel fully alive. On page 70 we give you a High Life Ten-Day Programme which can be followed as a short-term, quick-fix regime to enhance your overall health. More significantly, the diet can be used as the blueprint for a permanent change in the way you eat to build and sustain optimum well-being.

The Big Idea

There is nothing complicated about High Life – just a few simple principles that determine what to eat and when to eat it. Breakfast is raw juice with green supplements and as much whole fruit as you want. Try to make lunch the main meal of the day. It begins with a green drink and is built around a terrific Trio Salad (see p. 131) composed of one root vegetable, one fruit vegetable, and one leafy vegetable. What else? A good source of protein such as tofu, eggs, steamed or grilled fish or chicken – preferably cooked without the skin – and organic meat.

Dinner should be light. Perhaps a glass of raw juice followed by a bowl of home-made vegetable soup spiked with sea vegetables for extra minerals and flavour, or a crunchy salad with some wholegrain bread.

It may not be practicable for you to take a long break in the middle of the day, but whenever possible make lunch your largest meal. This is when you most need energy for the day.

If you get into the habit of eating light in the evening, you'll find that you will sleep far better at night. Soon, you will probably find that you are sleeping a lot less, too. When your body is detoxified and functioning efficiently, you will sleep more soundly. Because the sleep you get on the High Life diet is more restful, you need less of it.

Cut out Coffee

We love coffee, adore the stuff. The kind of coffee we particularly like is real strong, dark and potent espresso of the kind that gives you a better buzz than amphetamine sulphate. The comparison with an illegal drug is apposite, since trimethyl xanthine – caffeine – is also habit-forming and its overuse can lead to headaches, insomnia, nervousness, and anxiety. Like speed, coffee gives you a quick lift and the illusion of energy, only to let you crash a few hours later in need of another caffeine injection to keep going. Consequently, while we still drink coffee occasionally, we're careful not to let it become a daily habit.

Have you ever had to work late, perhaps revising for an exam, and kept yourself going with endless cups of coffee? If so, you'll be familiar with that wired mental state in which your thoughts are racing, but you just can't seem to get them into any sort of comprehensible order. Caffeine stimulates your nervous system and makes you feel alert, but tests have demonstrated that in reality the drug causes confusion and nervousness. Rather than help you concentrate, too much coffee has the effect of disconnecting you from your instincts and, in extreme cases, can provoke a psychotic reaction. In fact, if you need a clear head and the stamina to keep studying for hours on end, the best thing to keep you going is a glass of raw juice.

Some people use coffee as a laxative, but while it's certainly effective at moving the bowels, caffeine has a strongly adverse effect on the digestive system as a whole. Tea is not much better for you. Even if you've always been a committed tea drinker, after a couple of weeks of living the Juice High life you'll find you don't miss it. Then, you will appreciate an occasional cup of Rosie Lee or powerful shot of espresso as one of life's simple pleasures rather than a matter of addiction.

Table Manners

Eating and drinking are usually seen as correlated activities. We tend to do both at meal times, simultaneously, sluicing chewed food down our oesophagus with abandon while raising the next forkful to our lips. Too often we eat on the run, cramming food into our mouths and washing it down with great gulps of drink. We know that eating like this isn't very dignified and probably isn't too good for the digestion, but we do it anyway. Then, when we get indigestion, we complain that there must have been something wrong with the food rather than the way we consumed it.

To live the High Life, however, you are going to have to do something about sloppy table manners. The High Life Diet requires you to become more discriminating about what you eat, and you must also be more fastidious about the way you eat it. While we occasionally enjoy a glass of wine or two over dinner, drinking a lot at meal times is not a good idea – for two reasons. First, drinking tends to make you chew your food less thoroughly than you should. Second, fluids dilute the saliva in your mouth and the gastric juices in your stomach, rendering them ineffective at breaking down the improperly chewed food.

Accompany your meals with a glass of spring water if you wish, but just the one. Sip it slowly between mouthfuls, to clear your palate. Take the time to chew your food thoroughly before swallowing it. Don't talk with your mouth full and don't leap up from the table as soon as you're finished, but take a calm minute to let your food settle.

Just Juice

You'll notice how a glass of raw juice tends to fill you up, as if it were a meal in itself. In fact, considering the nutritional value of raw juice, it *is* a meal in itself and should be consumed on its own. Raw juice is easy to digest, but it still has to pass through your stomach to be assimilated in your intestines and anything eaten at the same time will only slow its passage. If taken on an empty stomach, raw juice will take no more than 20 minutes to pass through your stomach. Therefore, make it a rule not to eat or drink anything for at least that length of time after downing a glass of raw juice.

The living enzymes in raw juice assist the digestion process and the neutralising effect of raw juice upon the internal environment of your body will provide the ideal conditions for food to be properly digested. Consequently, raw juice makes the ideal aperitif, or first course of a meal. At dinner parties, your guests will be delighted and amazed by being offered a glass of freshly-extracted raw juice in place of the soup. Just remember (and tell your friends!) to sip your juice slowly, mixing it with the saliva in your mouth, and try to wait half an hour before moving on to the main course.

With fruit juices, the half hour rule is slightly different, but even more important. Fruit juices pass through your stomach really quickly, in 10 or 15 minutes, so long as there is no food in the way. If the exit to your intestines is blocked by half-digested food, the fruit juice will be trapped in your stomach where it will start to ferment, causing bloating and flatulence. For this reason, fresh fruit and fruit juices should only be consumed on an empty stomach. In order to allow your body to complete its work of elimination before you start to burden your system once more with food, resolve to consume nothing but freshly-extracted fruit juices right up until midday.

One Green Glass

Fruit juices are fabulous, naturally, and we have yet to meet someone who wasn't beguiled by their first taste of Carrot & Apple. These are the easiest juices to accept, but they are far from being the most beneficial. In Chapter Seven, we explain more about the amazing and as yet unexplained but awesomely powerful health-promoting factors in the juices of green, leafy vegetables. To really live the High Life, you must incorporate more green vegetables into your diet. That's not a radical statement; everybody is saying it, from Government agencies to your mum.

To derive the maximum benefit from your juicer, therefore, you must make full use of the pungent and powerfully-flavoured dark green juices extracted from such vegetables as spinach, broccoli and cabbage. These all contain an abundance of micro-nutrients, enzymes and trace elements that are easily denatured by heat and totally destroyed by cooking. By juicing them, we are able to extract most of the essential goodness of raw vegetables and supply our bodies with unadulterated, natural green nutrition.

The snag is that these green juices tend to be something of an acquired taste. They are too strong to be drunk straight and must be diluted with blander and more watery salad vegetables, like cucumber and celery. Cucumbers are rich in minerals, but are mostly water; the juice is a strong diuretic and the best skin toner we know of. Unfortunately, the bright green specimens you see in the supermarket have often been sprayed with pesticides and waxed to preserve their appeal. Unless you're sure your cuke is organic, peel it. Celery has a mildly salty flavour and is also good for the complexion. It's often a bit muddy at the root, so wash each stalk thoroughly before you put it through the juicer.

Make it a rule that you will drink at least one glass of green juice each day. That doesn't mean you have to stick exclusively to green ingredients, just make sure that they form a good percentage of what you juice. Use a base of carrot and apple, as we do in the Raw NRG mix (see p. 124) and gradually include more and more green, as in the More Raw NRG cocktail (see p. 38). Generally speaking, the darker green the colour of your juice, the more good it's going to do you.

Less is More

Busy people tend to skip meals. They get caught up in their work, rushing to meet deadlines, and neglect to eat. This is by no means a bad thing, since being slightly hungry tends to make us more alert and creative. In fact it would be fine if, once their work was done, these busy people took their time to prepare and consume a properly-balanced meal like the ones we suggest in the Recipe section (see pages 131–136). But busy people don't tend to do that. They're too busy. So they live on convenience food.

People who want to lose weight in a hurry also tend to skip meals. They think that by doing without lunch they can forgo a few calories and maybe shed a few ounces. It might work, too, except that too often they find them-

selves craving confectionery in the middle of the afternoon, or being irresistibly drawn to the soft drinks
machine in the corner of the office. There's nothing
wrong with skipping meals, so long as you don't try to
compensate for the meal you missed by eating (or drinking) junk later on.

Not only is there nothing wrong with skipping meals,
it can be positively good for you. Increasingly, scientific
evidence suggests that longevity can be significantly
increased by a diet that contains a high level of essential
nutrients, but about a third fewer calories than are
conventionally thought necessary to maintain 'normal'
body weight. A glass of raw juice is the ultimate dietary
supplement and the perfect replacement for a bulky
meal because it is nutrient-dense, but calorie-lean.
Have a glass of raw juice instead of lunch and you will
probably have plenty of energy to last you through until
teatime. If you miss lunch and come home starving,
don't dive into the biscuit barrel or raid the fridge for
something to snack on before dinner. Make yourself a
glass of raw juice instead.

Where's the Fibre?

Nutritionally, raw juice is excellent, but it is deficient in
one department. Of all the insoluble fibre contained
within the fruits and vegetables you juice, none of it goes
into the glass. It's precisely because all the fibre has been
extracted that raw juice is so effective in delivering essential nutrients to the body, but mankind cannot live by
juice alone. Plenty of fibre in your diet is a prerequisite
for good health and proper elimination, because it provides the muscles in your digestive tract with something
solid to work with and acts as a peristaltic broom, collect-
ing faecal matter in your colon and propelling it to the
bowels. Fibre, as they say, keeps you regular.

The best source of fibre is raw fruits and vegetables,
whole grains and pulses, of which you'll find plenty in

the High Life Diet. Raw juice does contain *some* soluble dietary fibre, but all the insoluble cellulose fibre ends up with the pulp. We're frequently asked what to do with the pulp left over from juicing and there are various ways in which it can be used.

Pulp Facts

Many of the books on juicing don't tell you what to do with the pulp. The pulp is important. The average person on a Western diet gets only 10–25 grammes of fibre a day, whereas our ancestors were used to 35–60 grammes a day, so the more fibre you can use from your juicing the better.

There are all sorts of things you can do with vegetable and fruit pulps, but there is one principle you have to know. Either use the pulp right away in whatever dish you want to make – salad, sorbet, meat loaf, sauce, or a poultice (more about this in a minute) – or freeze it. It is easy to freeze fruit and vegetable pulps in plastic bags which you can then use at your leisure.

Cheap Beauty

There are all sorts of wonderful external poultices you can make from vegetable and fruit pulps. The pulps of kiwi fruit, pineapple, papaya and mango are wonderful for refining skin – in fact they are the natural source of the AHA fruit acids that you pay a fortune for in expensive skin creams. Simply apply the pulp to your skin, leave it on for ten minutes and rinse off. Because these tropical fruits contain proteolytic enzymes they will quite literally digest the dead skin cells on the surface of your skin, leaving it smoother, fresher, and regenerated.

The pulp from potatoes and cucumber are very useful as eye compresses. Simply place between two pieces of cheesecloth or cotton and lay over your closed eyelids while you rest for ten or fifteen minutes. This takes away bags from under the eyes, and minimises black circles.

Pumpkin, cucumber, carrot and marrow pulps are great for calming skin inflammations, whether they be eczema rash or sunburn. They are very cooling to the body and can be useful when you have a mild fever. Place in a compress in between two pieces of cotton on the forehead or just over the liver.

Pulps make great additions to salads too. You can also use pulp to stuff courgettes, tomatoes, marrows, even twice-baked potatoes. (Bake a potato, take out the inner part of the potato, mix with vegetable pulp, season with salt, pepper, and a little olive oil. Put back in the oven, sprinkled with some chopped spring onions, and rebake for fifteen minutes.) Pulp also goes well in pasta salads. And you can make wonderful soups by juicing vegetables, then mixing some of the juice back into the pulp and eating it immediately.

Delicious Sweets

You can use the pulp of fruits to bake beautiful sweet breads and rolls or to make carrot cake. Fruit pulps, fresh or frozen, such as apricot, pear, apple and peach, are great things to add to porridge, muesli or cereals along with a dash of cinnamon, nutmeg or cardamom. They bring a natural sweetness to the cereal without your ever having to add honey or sugar. You can also mix fruit pulps with yoghurt, cottage cheese or tofu, adding a little unsulphured blackstrap molasses or maple syrup to make delicious shakes. Finally, you can use fruit pulps warmed up a little to make delicious toppings for toast, pancakes or muffins. You can even mix them in with minced lamb or beef, pork or chicken, to make delicious high-fibre patties. Any pulp left over that you don't have a use for makes fabulous compost. You don't even have to wait for it to rot down; just spread it around your garden.

Here are a few of our favourite pulp recipes but do develop your own. You would be surprised how much you can get out of pulp.

Coleslaw

2 cups cabbage pulp
2 cups carrot pulp
1 cup apple pulp
1 tbsp cider vinegar

3 tbsp olive oil
2 tbsp chopped parsley
A handful of chopped spring
    onions

Mix all the pulps together, stir in the vinegar and
olive oil and garnish with the parsley and spring
onion.

Pasta Salad

1 bag wholegrain pasta of your
    choice
3 tbsp carrot pulp
3 tbsp celery pulp
3 tbsp tomato pulp

3 tbsp cauliflower pulp
salt and pepper to taste
1 tsp oregano
2 squeezed cloves garlic
4 tbsp olive oil

Cook the pasta and chill. Add the rest of the ingredients, mix and serve.

Yummy Carrot Cake

1 cup cold-pressed sesame
    oil or olive oil
3 cups carrot pulp
1 cup apple pulp
1 cup honey
1/2 cup blackstrap
    molasses

1 tsp pure vanilla extract
3 eggs
3 cups wholegrain flour
1 1/2 tsp baking soda
2 tsp nutmeg
1 cup raisins

Mix the pulps and oil together, add the honey,
molasses, vanilla and eggs and mix together well. Sift
together the dry ingredients and add to the mixture,
stir until blended. Add the raisins, pour into an oiled
baking pan and bake for one hour at 180°C (350°F)
Gas 4.

Blueberry Muffins

3 cups carrot pulp
1½ cups pineapple pulp
1 cup honey
3 eggs
1 cup cold-pressed sesame
    oil or extra-virgin olive
    oil

1 tbsp vanilla
3 cups wholegrain flour
1 tbsp baking soda
1 tsp nutmeg
1½ cups fresh or frozen whole
    blueberries

Mix the carrot and the pineapple pulp together, add the honey, eggs, oil and vanilla and mix. Sift together the dry ingredients and add to the mixture. Add the blueberries and stir in gently. Pour into muffin papers or greased muffin tins. Bake for 45 minutes at 180°C (350°F) Gas 4.

Pulp Sorbet

Collect about three cups of pulp from any sweet fruit – peaches, apples, cherries, pears, apricots, pineapple, raspberries, strawberries. Freeze in an ice-cube tray and when frozen put into a food processor with 4 ripe bananas and blend to the consistency of sorbet. Serve immediately.

Fruit Sauce

Take 1 cup of pulp from any sweet fruit, blend together with 2tbsp honey or organic maple syrup and serve on toast or pancakes or over ice cream.

Total Juicing

Conventional juicers, whether they be centrifugal juicers or extruding juicers, all separate the juice from the pulp. You then have the option of using the pulp (which is what we strongly recommend since it is full of vitamins and minerals) or throwing it away. However, there is a whole new approach to juicing which is worth getting into. It is called molecular juicing, or *total juicing*, and it requires a totally different piece of equipment from the machine you use for ordinary juice making.

Total juicing is a way of juicing the entire vegetable or fruit, from which you discard nothing. It actually pulverises the fruit or vegetable to such a fine degree that you are able to absorb the nutrients almost immediately. This form of juicing is wonderful for anyone who has a digestive problem, for babies, for anyone who wants to get large quantities of fibre – for example, someone who is slimming – and for anyone whose digestion is less than perfect.

For total juicing you need a very strong machine. Conventional blenders are not capable of molecular or total juicing. They will give you a mush that is highly unpleasant. You need to remember that total juicing takes a lot more skill in what you mix with what, as if you mix combinations of fruits and vegetables together indiscriminately you can end up with a mess that tastes disgusting.

Total juicing is also a wonderful way of increasing the fibre in your diet. Many important ingredients in a fruit or vegetable are actually left in the fibre (and that's another reason why we urge you strongly not to discard the pulp). For instance, when you extract the juice from an orange you get approximately 30IU of beta-carotene, but 30 more are discarded in the pulp. With a carrot, you get 14,000IU of carotene in the juice but another 9800IU remain in the fibre. With total juicing you get them all.

The juice you produce by placing your fruits or vegetables cut into convenient sized pieces into a molecular or total juicer is not as sweet as that which is extracted from one of the more conventional juicers. Hence total juicers can be a good thing for people with blood sugar problems, since occasionally they may find that the sweetness of carrot and apple, for instance, is such that it stimulates the pancreas to produce too much insulin.

Total juices have a thicker, smoother texture, a totally different feeling in the mouth to the juices which come out of ordinary juice extractors. Occasionally you might find you want to add a little sweetening to total juices and this is best done in the form of maple syrup or natural unheated honey. You will probably also need to add a little water or some ice cubes in order to give a bit more liquid for the pulverising process to take place properly.

Soups & Sprouts

If you have a blender capable of total juicing, first make your vegetable or fruit juice in the ordinary way and then use it as an additive in your total juicing. So, if you have made some carrot juice, use it as a base for making beautiful vegetable soups (see Recipes, pages 134–136). Similarly you can use fruit juices as a base for making fruit frappés by mixing together whole fruits – peaches, apricots, berries – in the blender with the juice that you have made from your conventional juicer.

Total juicing is a great way of using sprouted alfalfa and mung beans. You simply take any vegetable or fruit juice, pour it into your total juicer and add a handful of your sprouts. Blend and drink immediately. The fibre in sprouted seeds is wonderful and it's a great way of getting the very best of both ways of juicing.

A total juicer is thus an ideal way of making green drinks. After preparing a vegetable or fruit juice in an ordinary juicer, pour into the blender and add green supplements such as fresh green beetroot leaves, kale, spinach or dandelion. You can also use the same method to add powdered wheat or barley grass to fresh juices. We always try to use organic fruits and vegetables for juicing just to be sure that we are protected from any intake of pesticides or herbicides.

HIGH LIFE TEN-DAY PROGRAMME

Now let's see what High Life looks like. Here are the basic guidelines for ten days to reorientate your eating habits permanently.

- Have juice for breakfast plus a green supplement either on its own or together with some fruit.

- Remember to *chew your juices and drink your food*. In other words, sip your juices slowly so they have a chance to mix with the saliva in the mouth to get the full benefit of everything that is in them, and chew your foods, until they turn into liquids.

- Avoid eating between meals since this slows down the stomach's emptying and encourages food that is still in the stomach to ferment, as well as creating false appetite. If you are hungry have a glass of fresh juice or lots of spring water between meals.

- Try to leave four to five hours between meals. This is the time your body needs in order to efficiently and completely digest its previous meal.

- Make meal times a pleasure.

- Drink as much water as you like, virtually the more the better. But don't drink water with meals – give yourself twenty minutes water-free before a meal and half an hour afterwards.

- Try to take your main meal at lunch and the light meal in the evening. This is an ideal way to live since you sleep much deeper and better if you don't eat heavily at night. However, you must suit your eating to your lifestyle and when you have to have a main meal at night, enjoy it.

A DAY ON THE HIGH LIFE DIET

Begin the day with a cup of hot or cold spring water with the juice of half a lemon and a little honey or organic maple syrup if desired.

Throughout the day drink as much spring water as you like. If you are hungry between meals have another glass of juice, preferably green.

Breakfast

Large glass fresh raw fruit juice – apple, orange, grape, grapefruit etc, or a recipe of your choice. To this add either some green leaves such as dandelion, beetroot, spinach, the juice from one of the cereal grasses, or a teaspoon to a tablespoon of one of the cereal grass supplements such as green barley, stirred into your glass of juice. You can drink more than one juice (with or without the extra green) and you can also have a piece of fruit or a bunch of grapes and as much herb tea as you like, sweetened with a little honey or maple syrup.

Main Meal

If at all possible make this meal at lunchtime since you will digest your food better and sleep better if you eat light in the evening. Large glass of fresh, raw vegetable juice, choose any mixture you like – carrot, raw beetroot, celery, cucumber, cabbage, tomato, spinach etc – or one of the recipes on pages 112–130.

A big salad – ideally one of the Trio Salads (see Recipes) together with some grilled fish, lamb's liver, free-range chicken, game, a tofu dish or an omelette.

Steamed or wok-fried vegetables.

Herb tea or coffee substitute.

Light Meal

Glass of fresh vegetable or fruit juice. A salad or light soup. Several slices of wholegrain bread or a bowl of live muesli. Herb tea or coffee substitute.

Chapter Six
Quick Fix

Because raw juice is the richest available source of vitamins, minerals and enzymes it is the best possible tonic for promoting all-round health and general well-being. Most people who embrace the Juice High lifestyle find that the minor complaints that used to irritate them fade away as the body rebalances itself and they become accustomed to feeling perfectly fine, all of the time. The key to building and sustaining an indomitable physiology, one which is strong, focused and invulnerable to illness, is the consumption of the broadest possible range of juices. However, each juice has specific therapeutic properties and this chapter shows how you can use raw juice to treat a range of common complaints.

Modern medical science tends to have a nuts and bolts approach in prescribing drugs to treat the symptoms of illness, frequently without paying attention to the underlying causes of the condition. Natural health practitioners try to take a holistic view, seeing the body as a complete organism with many parts, all of which must operate synergistically for the whole being to be healthy. Illness is the result of disharmony, or a chemical imbalance in the body caused by nutritional deficiency.

Here are our suggestions as to which foods you should eat (and which ones you should avoid) in order to alleviate the misery of a number of all-too-common complaints. Our suggestions are followed, in each case, by a list of appropriate juice recipes that you'll find in the Recipe Section which begins on page 112. Most of the conditions described below will respond rapidly when you drink the recommended juices, but do remember that these are only recommendations, not prescriptions. Any attempt to treat a medical condition should always come under the direction of a competent physician.

Acne

A lot of acne is the result of eating a diet high in sugar and low in fibre. When the body is not eliminating waste properly, the pores of the skin become blocked. It is very important to make sure that you eat plenty of vegetables that are rich in fibre (not wheat or wheat bran as in wholegrain bread as this tends to clog up people who suffer from acne and skin problems). Steer clear of processed convenience foods (they are full of the kind of hydrogenated fats you find in margarines) and stick to using olive oil for your salads and wok frying. Do a detox and use the High Life Diet, emphasising the fresh vegetables and fruits. Avoid dairy products.

Carrot juice is very beneficial for acne, but the green juices are supreme. Drink lots and lots of fresh carrot juice, to which you add as much green as you can manage, as often as you can manage it. The best sources of green are cabbage and kale, beetroot and turnip tops, watercress and spinach, parsley and dandelion leaves.

Carrot & Apple	*Ginger Spice*
Carrot High	*Green Friend*
Chlorophyll Plus	

Allergy

All allergies, from the classic antibody antigen reactions that cause the release of histamine, to food allergies which can act quite differently, must be treated holistically. That means diet, rest, stress management and the elimination of any possible trigger foods or environmental chemicals.

Sugar is the first thing that needs to be eliminated completely from the diet. Cut out packaged convenience foods that are full of additives such as aspartamine – the sulphites in prepared meat foods – and monosodium glutamate (MSG). Many allergic people have an over-growth of candida albicans yeast in their bodies and need to address this at the same time. Milk products are best avoided by anyone with any sort of allergic condition.

Most allergic reactions occur when the body is over-acidic. A high alkaline diet, such as a Raw Energy-type regime, plus lots of alfalfa sprouts or juice (which is rich in mineral salts) can help to create the right internal environment. Celery will also help you become allergy-free. Grapefruit, orange, cantaloupe and parsley are rich in the bioflavonoids; spinach, kale and sweet peppers are rich in B6, which can be particularly helpful for many sensitivities; garlic, spinach and cauliflower are a good source of molybdenum, a trace element that tends to be deficient in people who are sensitive to the sulphites and MSG.

Celery Sticks	*Red Cool*
Parsley Passion	*Sprout Special*

Anaemia

Anaemia occurs either when there is a decrease in the total number of red blood cells, or in the volume of the blood, or when red blood cells become abnormal in shape or size. This condition tends to make you pale and weak and inhibits your resistance to infection. It often creates insomnia, leading to irritability and depression and causing chronic fatigue. There are a number of different underlying deficiencies that are present when one is anaemic; iron is important in order to be able to form new red blood cells, and folic acid and vitamin B12 help to rebuild red blood cells. If anaemia persists, consult your doctor. It could possibly be the result of abnormalities in the production of haemoglobin itself.

Green drinks and green foods are essential for anaemia sufferers. They are rich in folic acid and many of them are rich in iron, particularly watercress, spinach, beetroot tops, dandelion leaves and the brassicas.

Vegetables which are particularly beneficial include parsley, green pepper, beetroot tops, carrot, kale, spinach and asparagus. Berries can be very useful, particularly for women (they are good for menstrual cramps, morning sickness and calming labour pains, not to mention sea sickness, yeast infections and poor circulation).

Try to drink as many green drinks as possible. To each glass add a teaspoon of spirulina, which is extremely rich in B12, and shake or blend well.

Beet Treat	*Easy Does It*
Dandelion Plus	*Green Zinger*
Double Whammy	*Red Flag*

Arthritis

Both osteoarthritis and rheumatoid arthritis have been successfully treated with juice therapy, which is particularly beneficial if the patient has not been on long-term drug treatment. Osteoarthritis affects the bones and joints with symptoms such as swelling of soft tissues, local tenderness, restricted movement, bony swellings and crackings of the joints as well as stiffness after resting. The more the joint is used in osteoarthritis, the worse the pain generally becomes. Rheumatoid arthritis produces inflammatory conditions in the joints and the structures surrounding joints, as well as a feeling of weakness, often with low-grade fever, long-term fatigue, pain and stiffness. Rheumatoid arthritis is increasingly considered an auto-immune reaction where the body has actually developed antibodies against its own tissues.

In both osteo- and rheumatoid arthritis, certain things are essential. Firstly, that you cut out foods from the nightshade family such as potatoes, aubergine, tomatoes, and peppers. Secondly (in the case of osteoarthritis) that you avoid citrus fruits such as limes, lemons, oranges and grapefruits. In the tradition of natural medicine these are believed to contribute to the inflammation.

With both forms of arthritis, it is important to avoid all convenience foods and refined foods such as white sugar, white flour, processed foods that contain chemical additives, and alcohol. Consider the possibility that you might have some sort of a sensitivity or allergic reaction to food, perhaps to wheat or to dairy products. Try eliminating wheat flour and everything made from it as well as all dairy products from your diet for three weeks and see if it makes a significant difference. In the case of rheumatoid arthritis it can be useful, if you are not a vegetarian, to eat more cold water fish such as tuna, sardines, salmon and mackerel which contain the essential fatty acid known as omega-3. Many people with arthritis fare better on a low-fat vegetarian diet.

Vegetables to incorporate into your juices include carrot, beetroot tops, broccoli, turnip, grapes, kale, cabbage, all dark green vegetables, apple, and ginger. Pineapple is particularly good for rheumatoid arthritis since it contains the enzyme bromelin which has anti-inflammatory properties.

Dandelion juice is excellent, especially for rheumatoid arthritis. Pick the dandelion greens carefully, from places which are not likely to have been sprayed and are not along the verges of roads where they may have picked up heavy metals such as lead from air pollution. Cut off the leaves and wash them well before putting them through the juicer. If you are used to drinking green juices you can actually drink dandelion juice on its own, or mixed equally with carrot. It also mixes well with a little watercress. If you are not used to drinking green juices, it can be useful to start with a delicious sweet juice such as carrot and apple and then gradually increase the levels of dandelion you are putting into it. Dandelion also has the ability to create an amazing high once the juice is assimilated into the liver, which usually takes about half an hour. But go easy, for if your digestive system is not used to green juices this can be too much of a shock. Start with small amounts and increase gradually.

Ginger Berry	*Popeye Punch*
Green Goddess	*Red Genius*
Green Wow	*Sprouting o' the Green*
Pineamint	*Top of the Beet*
Pineapple Green	

Asthma

The theory is that asthma comes in two forms. One kind is said to be caused by specific allergens either in the air or food; the other is said to have no particular cause. Most experts in natural medicine, however, find that there is always an allergic element, as there is also always an emotional one in any kind of asthma or other condition in which the symptoms include spasms of the bronchial tubes and swelling of the mucous membrane.

Perhaps the most important remedy is to eliminate from the diet any foods that create mucus in the body. This means not eating dairy products, coffee, tea, chocolate, wheat, and convenience foods. Many asthmatics find they do best when they eliminate from their diet not only wheat but other grains as well (except for buckwheat, which is not a true grain, and brown rice or millet). Asthmatics seem to be more affected by food allergies than other people, which can result in inflammation of the bronchial tubes that causes an even stronger reaction to smoke, pollen and air pollutants such as sulphur-dioxide. Asthma also appears to weaken the adrenal glands, so handling it means living on a low-allergy diet in which at least 50 per cent of the foods that you eat are taken raw.

Juices that are rich in magnesium, which relaxes the bronchial muscle, are particularly useful, including turnip, watercress, kale, turnip greens, parsley, collard greens, carrots, asparagus and beetroot tops. A couple of tablespoons of lemon juice added to any glass of fresh raw juice is a traditional treatment for asthma, as are molasses, which can be a useful additive to a glass of any juice. Other additives which are equally useful include fresh ginger, onions, and garlic (in small quantities, if you wish to keep your friends).

Carrot High	*Hi NRG*
Glorious Grapefruit	*Leslie's Cocktail*
Hi Mag	*Potassium Punch*

Cellulite

Orange peel skin – the lumps and bumps that are so hard to get rid of, even in slim women – can be shed provided you take a total body approach to the issue. Women with cellulite are often constipated, even if they have one bowel movement a day, and they also tend to have poor lymphatic drainage, so that wastes are not eliminated properly. In addition, many women with cellulite suffer from poor liver function and an under-active thyroid.

Foods that are rich in bioflavonoids such as sweet peppers, tomatoes, cabbage, parsley and citrus fruits (incorporate the pithy, white covering inside the peel in your juices) are important because they help strengthen the capillaries so you don't get leakage and the pockets of water that create *peau d'orange* flesh. Vitamin C is also important to strengthen the capillaries, as is zinc. If you want to shed cellulite permanently, shift the percentage of raw foods in your diet so that you are consuming between 50 and 75 per cent of your foods raw. Use skin brushing, cut out *all* convenience foods which are replete with junk fats and chemicals, and eliminate coffee and tea.

Remember that cellulite is slow to form and slow to clear, but it *will* go away provided you are persistent. These juices will be beneficial:

Ginger Berry	*Pineapple Green*
Ginger's Best	*Potassium Power*
Hi Mag	*Waterfall*

Colds

The common cold has for generations been considered by natural health practitioners to be the body's means of eliminating waste when it has become overloaded. When you feel yourself coming down with a cold eliminate all dairy products from your diet and all foods with sugar in them. Do a Juice Blitz and follow that by following the High Life Diet for at least a week.

Juicing for colds has two goals. The first is to strengthen the immune system, and for this you need lots of greens – kale, parsley, green pepper, watercress – which contain plenty of anti-oxidants such as beta-carotene (don't forget your carrots too) as well as vitamin C, chlorophyll and all of those as yet unexplained plant properties which are so strengthening to the body. The second purpose of juicing for colds is in many ways the most important and that is elimination. This means using juices from vegetables and fruits which help eliminate waste from the system. These include lemon, apricot, garlic, parsley, ginger, watercress, kale, radish, spinach, apple, pear and tomato.

Atomic Lift-Off	*Hi Mag*
Beetroot, Carrot &	*Pineapple Grapefruit Drink*
Orange	*Red Genius*
Carrot High	*Salad Juice*
Ginger Spice	*Sweet and Spicy*

Constipation

Constipation is the hidden condition that, according to natural health practitioners, is so widespread that it would be hard to quantify it. These experts insist that very few of us are actually cleansing our colon as thoroughly as we should. Most people find that when they begin to take juices and eat a higher percentage of their foods raw, their constipation clears by itself and they begin to have two or three bowel movements a day. It is essential to overall health that the bowels function really well, for if faecal matter stays in the colon then harmful substances from the natural bacteria that live in the bowel can contribute to the development of many specific ailments such as haemorrhoids, varicose veins, hernias, cellulite, flatulence, obesity, insomnia, bad breath, indigestion and diverticulitis. Constipation also plays a part in the development of degenerative diseases, from cancer to coronary heart disease, diabetes and even long-term depression.

One of the best natural remedies for constipation is rhubarb. Rhubarb is a vegetable but is usually thought of as a fruit. It is rich in calcium, phosphorus, iron, sodium, potassium, vitamin A, folic acid, vitamin C and magnesium. Raw rhubarb, like spinach, also contains oxalic acid, which you don't want to get too much of. Therefore rhubarb is not an ingredient we would use daily in any of our juices. Rhubarb is useful for intestinal parasites and for intestinal wind, and rhubarb juice applied externally is traditionally used to treat leg ulcers, bed sores and wounds. However, rhubarb juice and spinach juice should not be taken by anyone who suffers from kidney stones, because of their high oxalic acid content.

Getting over constipation is usually a simple matter once you begin to juice, but there are a number of juices that are especially useful during the transition stage. Rhubarb, apples, spinach, prunes and pears all have a natural laxative effect.

Apples & Pears	*Ginger's Best*
Beet Treat	*Rhubarb Radiance*
Black Watermelon	*Spinapple*
Carrot, Beet, Celery,	*Sprout Special*
Tomato	*Tropical Prune*

Depression

Feeling depressed is not just a psychological condition. Very often that sense of purposelessness, emptiness, feelings of worthlessness and guilt, come from a biochemical imbalance in the body. Internal pollution is a major cause, which is why a Juice Blitz plus a week on the High Life Diet shifts depression for many people.

Sugar and caffeine should be avoided and it is important to check for any food allergies. Nobody who is depressed should be eating convenience foods, even those so-called comfort foods that are supposed to cheer us up. The neurotransmitters – hormones in the brain which control feeling – are derived from the food we eat, so the food has got to be good. Serotonin (derived from the amino acid tryptophan) is a particularly significant neurotransmitter. When there are adequate levels of serotonin in the brain the mood tends to be elevated and sleep normal; low serotonin levels are associated with mood distortions and interrupted sleep patterns. A meal rich in complex carbohydrates helps the body absorb tryptophan, and therefore promotes the production of serotonin.

Bananas, figs and dates are rich in tryptophan. Carbohydrate in the form of a piece of toast and a banana before bed can help tremendously to induce sleep and also create a sense of calm peacefulness (provided, of course, that you are not allergic to the grains from which the toast is made).

To banish the blues permanently, increase the levels of raw food in your diet to between 50 and 75 per cent each day. Try using the Juice Blitz one day each week for a few weeks as well, to help continue the detoxification process. Meanwhile make your juices rich in dark green vegetables full of magnesium, potassium, iron, calcium and folic acid. A deficiency in any of these can contribute to depression, as can a deficiency in fatty acids, which is why it can be useful to add linseeds to your juices. Don't be discouraged if it takes a little time to deep-cleanse your body and replenish the nutrients you may be lacking. It is well worth the effort.

Chlorophyll Plus   *Pineamint*
Ginger Spice   *Red Genius*
Hi Mag   *Salsa Surprise*
Linusit Perfect

Digestion

Digestive troubles come in many forms, from minor problems such as a bloated feeling after a meal, to abdominal pain and wind, nausea, and more serious ailments like gastric ulcers, diverticulitis, and colon troubles. In all these circumstances, it's important to avoid taking in any substances that can irritate the gut, such as coffee, alcohol and chocolate. Occasionally stomach troubles come from *hypochlorhydria* – a deficiency of hydrochloric acid – in which case pineapple and papaya juice are excellent since they are rich in the protein-digesting enzymes bromelin and papain.

Among clinical reports of juicing, none is more impressive than the results that Dr Garnett Cheney of Stanford University reported for his treatment of gastric ulcers using juices alone. Dr Cheney prescribed for his patients fresh raw green cabbage juice, prepared and drunk immediately. It contains anti-peptic ulcer factors which have a really quite remarkable effect.

Leslie's mother, who was diagnosed with a peptic ulcer at the age of 37 and who was very resistant to taking any form of medication, read about Cheney's work and began to use cabbage juice. She drank about five 300ml (8oz) glasses a day for six weeks and then took smaller quantities for several months. The ulcers cleared up and she was never troubled by them again.

Cabbage juice tends to benefit most digestive upsets. It's not exactly delicious, however, and it can be helpful to mix it with pineapple juice to soften the flavour. Ginger is also good for digestion and has been used for thousands of years to counteract nausea, travel sickness, and morning sickness. Bananas have been shown to help protect the stomach from excess hydrochloric acid. Most people with any digestive upset that is not a serious medical condition requiring treatment find that simply getting into a Juice High way of living clears up the problem. The following juices are especially good for that purpose:

Gingeroo	*Red Flag*
Ginger Spice	*Red Genius*
Pineappage	*Tropical Prune*

Eczema

An annoying condition that's often hard to get rid of, where the skin becomes red, swollen and itchy in the beginning, then later thickens to produce crusted, scaly patches, eczema has many causes. Allergies are often a prime factor, which makes it important to use an elimination diet and to check for any food allergies. With eczema, as with any skin condition, it is important that your elimination works properly so that your skin is not forced to eliminate waste the hard way. Try the Juice Blitz and the High Life Diet.

Certain nutrients are also very important in the treatment of eczema. Sweet peppers, tomatoes, cabbage and parsley are all excellent sources of bioflavonoids, which help reduce inflammation and control allergy, as well as enhancing the capillary function so you get a better flow of nutrients and elimination of waste from the skin. Citrus fruits are also good, provided you incorporate the pithy, white covering inside the peel in your juices. Zinc is particularly important. It's usually found in good quantities in carrots, garlic, parsley, and ginger. Carrot and parsley are also prime sources of beta-carotene as are kale and spinach.

Carrot & Apple	*Green Wow*
Chlorophyll Plus	*Parsley Passion*
Gingeroo	*Spring Salad*

Eye Health

The health of the eyes depends more than anything else on the quality of anti-oxidant protection that your body gets. Free radical damage is a major factor in the development of both minor eye problems, such as short-sightedness, to major problems, such as cataracts and glaucoma. For the eye to remain healthy it needs to be able to maintain a normal balance and concentration of such minerals as calcium, potassium and sodium within the lens. When free radical damage occurs the cellular mechanisms by which nutrients are pumped to the eyes and excess sodium and wastes removed no longer work so well. Beta-carotene, one of the most important of all of the bioflavonoids, is an anti-oxidant that helps protect the eye lens from ultra-violet damage.

Yellow, orange and dark green vegetables which are rich in beta-carotene as well as vitamins C and E, the B complex, zinc, calcium and phosphorus are very important for eye health. Ginger, garlic and parsley are rich in zinc, another mineral element that has been shown to be helpful. There is anecdotal evidence that drinking lots of carrot juice will improve eye sight, particularly night vision. Here are some of our favourite recipes for eyes.

Beet Treat	*Hi Mag*
Carrot & Apple	*Orange Tonic*
Double Whammy	*Pineapple Green*
Green Wild	*Spiked Celery*

Fatigue

One of the underlying causes of fatigue, particularly in women, can be iron depletion. Spinach juice is a far better way of boosting iron levels than taking tablets, which tend to be highly constipating and are not really absorbed very well. The iron in natural foods and juices such as spinach, or any of the green leafy vegetables, and also in legumes, poultry, whole grains, liver and molasses, is highly bioavailable, i.e. your body has no trouble making use of it. Remember that replenishing the body with essential nutrients takes time and so be prepared to work with natural foods and juices for several weeks before you start to see lasting relief from chronic fatigue.

Again, make sure that 50–75 per cent of the foods you eat each day are raw and make sure you get lots of chlorophyll-rich foods. Cereal grasses are good, as they are high in minerals, vitamins and enzymes and also have a wonderful ability to enliven the liver and thereby to create more energy. Chlorophyll also helps protect from infectious diseases. You can take wheat and barley-grass juice as a supplement in powdered form that you add to your vegetables and fruit juices or you can go the whole hog and get a cereal grass juicer and grow your own cereal grasses (see Resources, p. 152).

Magnesium is another important mineral when it comes to fatigue. Low intracellular magnesium makes the body very prone to infection, food allergies and chronic conditions. Good sources of magnesium are any of the dark green vegetables, whole grains, seaweeds, molasses, legumes, fish and nuts.

Atomic Lift-Off	*Hi Mag*
Citrusucculent	*Hit the Grass*
Dandelion Plus	*Parsley Passion*
Ginger Berry	*Secret of the Sea*
Gingeroo	*Spinapple*
Glorious Grapefruit	*Sprout Special*
Green Zinger	

Hair Loss
You may be genetically programmed to lose your hair, but that doesn't mean you have to let it go easily. There is a great deal you can do to prevent hair loss and at the very least slow it down dramatically. Eat more foods that are rich in sulphur, amino acids, L-methionine and L-cysteine. Eggs are good, but cabbage is king.

Sugars will tend to increase the rate of hair loss so try to eliminate sugar completely from your diet. Include in your diet plenty of foods which are rich in PABA, inositol and choline, such as mushrooms, spinach, legumes, lentils, brown rice. Consider adding a supplement of vacuum-packed flaxseeds to your diet. You can grind them in a coffee grinder and sprinkle them on salads or cereals in the morning. You can also add them to your juices.

Finally, the grain alfalfa, particularly in its sprouted form, has long been believed to stimulate hair growth. Other juices for incipient slapheads include:

Alfalfa – Father of all	*Ginger's Best*
Juices	*Parsnip Perfect*
Carrot High	*Spinapple*
Fatty Acid Frolic	

Hangover

The inevitable consequence of over-indulgence is waking up feeling dehydrated and nauseous, with a brain that feels as if it's banging against the side of your head when you move. You need to replenish your bodily fluids, renutrify exhausted muscles and get your head together. Fruit juice is strongly indicated. Citrus juices, being full of natural sugar and vitamin C, are the most immediately effective remedy, but they may be a bit harsh if your stomach is delicate. Watermelon, being exceptionally mild, is ideal.

There is an art to hangover management and the key to it is regarding detoxification as the corollary of intoxication. All drugs provoke a strongly acidic reaction in the body which causes the symptoms of a hangover and the first step to recovery is to correct the body's chemical imbalance. Plain old Carrot & Apple juice is effective for re-balancing and it's easy to take when you're feeling weak. Beet juice will greatly assist the repair of any possible damage done to your liver and kidneys.

Apples & Pears	*Merry Belon*
Beet Treat	*Virgin Mary*
Carrot & Apple	

Insomnia

Insomnia can have many causes. Drugs such as beta blockers or thyroid medication, even caffeine and alcohol can all disrupt sleep. So, ironically, can sleeping pills, if your body becomes addicted to them.

Getting regular exercise – taking long walks rather than going to aerobics classes and throwing your back out of place – can help enormously to reduce the nervous tension that prevents sleep. Sometimes sleep is disrupted by hypoglycaemia, so make sure you don't have a blood sugar problem (see *Low Blood Sugar* below). Eliminate coffee, tea, alcohol and junk foods – including diet colas – from your life once and for all. Eat your biggest meal at lunchtime, as everyone sleeps better (and longer) when their stomach is not full. Consider using one of the well-proven natural tranquillisers such as Valerian, Passiflora (Passion flower) or Wild Lettuce. You can make a night-cap cocktail to help increase the levels of serotonin in the brain: blend a pinch of one of these natural tranquillisers into it.

Magnesium, vitamin B6 and niacin have to be present in order for the amino acid tryptophan to be able to turn itself into serotonin. Carrots are a rich source of all three. Calcium induces muscle relaxation and so does folic acid which in sufficient quantities prevents leg twitching and calms nervous tension. The green drinks, from dandelion to parsley and spinach, are excellent sources of folic acid and calcium. Seaweed is also a good source of magnesium. Many people (except those with low blood sugar) need an extra boost of fruit sugar before going to bed to trigger sleep. Pineapple and grape is a wonderful combination for this. Others include:

Green Goddess	*Smooth as Silk*
Hi Mag	*Spicy Carrot*
Lazy Lettuce	*Sprout Special*
Pineamint	

Low Blood Sugar (Hypoglycaemia)

Low blood sugar, where the body tends to secrete insulin which in turn makes the blood sugar level drop depriving the brain of its main 'food', glucose, is a condition that underlies much of the chocolate munching and coffee drinking that people indulge in in order to keep themselves going.

Hypoglycaemia involves disturbance to the balance of hormones in the body and can produce an enormous number of periodic symptoms including palpitations of the heart, sweating, depression, anxiety, headaches, poor concentration and bad temper. These symptoms are alleviated by munching on some sort of carbohydrate, such as a slice of wholegrain bread. The trick in clearing up the condition, however, is to clear out of your life everything that would trigger the pancreas to over-secrete insulin. In particular this means no sugar, chocolate, or bottled fruit juices. Choose foods that are rich in complex carbohydrates and fibre such as raw vegetables, whole oats, beans, wholegrain pasta, lentils, chick peas, etc. Sprouted seeds are particularly useful.

The vegetable juices are better than the fruit juices until blood sugar is stabilised. If you're hypoglycaemic, don't drink fruit juices unless they are well diluted with mineral water, and then only a couple of times a week. Try adding a little turmeric or cinnamon to your juices. Both these spices have long been used to help stabilise blood sugar. Foods which are rich in chromium will help regulate glucose metabolism in the body. These include spinach, apples, green peppers, whole grains, clams and liver. Use foods which are rich in manganese such as carrots, celery, beetroot, beetroot greens, turnip greens, pineapple, liver, eggs, green vegetables and buckwheat.

An antidote for a sweet tooth is lots of green drinks, but you will have to get yourself used to drinking them since they are about the last thing the hypoglycaemic wants. Once you do get used to it you will find that blood sugar stabilises and you have energy to spare, day in and day out. All of the green juices are excellent, such as:

Dandelion Plus	*Parsley Passion*
Green Friend	*Secret of the Sea*
Green Zinger	*Spicy Apple*
Lemon Zinger	*Tossled Carrot*

Migraine

When Leslie was 25 years old, she met a doctor who taught her about supporting the body to heal itself using juices and raw foods. Dr Philip Kilsby experienced 99 per cent success in the treatment of migraine, using juices, lots of raw fruits and vegetables, and a few dietary supplements. The only case of migraine he had not been able to cure was that of a woman who turned out not to have migraine but a brain tumour.

Kilsby taught that all migraine, regardless of cause, is centred in a liver that is over-worked trying to keep the body internally clear. So Kilsby took stress off the liver by removing from the diet foods that people are commonly allergic to such as red wine, other alcohol, salad cream, red plums, soft cheeses, figs, aged game, chicken liver, canned meat, salami sausages, pickled herring, aubergine, soy sauce and yeast concentrates, as well as chocolate, wheat, milk, the food colouring tartrazine, sugar, coffee and peanuts.

Kilsby then put his patients on a detox programme very much like the Juice Blitz, and followed it with a regime similar to the High Life Diet. Kilsby insisted his patients drink a juice rich in green vegetables twice daily. He found that his patients experienced migraines of decreasing intensity until, once their bodies were detoxified, the migraines altogether ceased.

Migraines result from contraction followed by rapid dilatation of the blood vessels in the brain, and this can be triggered by certain foods. Biofeedback can be help-ful: this involves training yourself to visualise your hands as warm, thereby drawing blood away from the head and taking pressure off the area that is involved in the migraine. The herb feverfew can also be useful to many people.

If you suffer from migraine banish all chemicals, including artificial sweeteners such as aspartamine, from your diet. Include in your juices some of the fruits and vegetables which are known to reduce platelet stickiness, since foods that inhibit blood clotting are known to reduce migraine. These include garlic, cantaloupe, and ginger.

Dandelion Plus   *Green Goddess*
Gingeroo   *Spring Salad*
Green Friend   *Sprout Special*

Prostate Trouble

Enlargement of the prostate is so common that 60 per cent of men between the ages of 40 and 59 have the condition, which is properly known as benign prostatic hyperplasia (BPH). When this occurs there is an obstruction of the bladder outlet, increased frequency of urination and difficulty in urinating. The standard medical treatment for BPH is surgery. However, there is a great deal that can be done to improve the condition through nutrition. BPH is a hormone-dependent disorder of the metabolism. Testosterone, especially free testosterone levels, decrease after the age of 55. Meanwhile levels of other hormones increase, particularly those of a very potent male hormone called dihydrotestosterone within the prostate itself which is responsible for the over-production of prostate cells. This ultimately results in the enlarged prostate.

Protecting yourself against high levels of xenoestrogens from the environment is an important part of diminishing prostate enlargement. You should also aim to reduce your stress levels, and to eliminate beer from your diet. The mineral zinc and vitamin B6 have been shown to have a beneficial effect: zinc, in particular, has been shown to reduce the size of the prostate and to reduce symptoms in men who suffer from BPH. Similarly, essential fatty acids such as those found in organic linseed or flaxseed oil have been shown to bring about a significant improvement in many patients with the condition.

It is important that sufferers from prostate trouble are protected as much as possible from pesticides, herbicides and other petrochemically derived compounds in the environment such as biphenyls, hexachlorobenzene and dioxin, which can increase the formation of dihydrotestosterone in the prostate. Go for juices that are high in zinc and B6 and drinks containing organically grown, vacuum-packed linseeds or flaxseeds.

Dandelion Plus	*Green Zinger*
Ginger's Best	*Linusit Perfect*
Ginger Spice	*Pineapple Green*
Green Friend	*Silky Strawberries*

Pre-Menstrual Syndrome

PMS comes in many forms and causes many symptoms, from irritability, depression, tension and decreased energy, to backache, breast pain, changes in libido, abdominal bloating, oedema and headache. There are certain things that all PMS sufferers need to watch. It is essential to clear sugar out of your diet as well as cut down on any other form of refined carbohydrates, including white flour and honey. Avoid coffee, tea and chocolate, for two reasons – first because they contain *methylxanthines*, which have been linked with a number of the symptoms associated with PMS, and secondly, because anything containing caffeine can have a very negative effect on such things as breast tenderness, anxiety and depression.

It is also a good idea to eliminate all milk products and wheat from your diet for seven days prior to menstruation. At the same time increase your intake of certain nutrients such as magnesium, B6 and the B complex, as well as beta-carotene. Bromelin too can be helpful since this enzyme is believed to help relax the smooth muscle tissue of the body. Go for the green juices, which are rich in all these things. If you have water retention, turn towards watermelon, grape, cucumber and dandelion, each of which has a splendid ability to eliminate excess water from the system. You are likely to find that all the juices that are good for PMS are also useful for someone who is wrestling with menopausal symptoms such as hot flushes. In both PMS and menopausal cases it can be helpful to follow a Raw Energy way of eating where 50–75 per cent of your foods are taken raw during the 7–10 days before a period or whenever the symptoms seem to be at their worst.

Black Watermelon	*Pineapple Special*
Cool as a Cuke	*Secret of the Sea*
Ginger Berry	*Spring Salad*
Green Zinger	*Sprout Special*
Hi Mag	*Waterfall*
Pineapple Green	

Stress
Stress is a complicated condition to treat as it has many causes and takes many forms. However, whenever the body is under prolonged stress the tissues tend to become more acidic. There is nothing better and more life-changing that you can do when your system is too acid than to drink fresh vegetable and fruit juices to alkalinise it. Detoxification helps eliminate the constant tension, anxiety and frustration that so often go with stress, as well its common consequences such as gastro-intestinal difficulties, high blood pressure, dizziness, loss of appetite or excessive appetite, and headaches.

While it is important to practise some sort of deep relaxation or meditation if you are suffering from prolonged stress, the effect of dietary change alone, incorporating a juice-high regime into your lifestyle and as always making between 50 and 75 per cent of your foods raw can literally transform your life within a fortnight. Useful nutrients include pantothenic acid, which occurs in good quantity in green leafy vegetables such as kale, dandelion and broccoli; potassium, which is found in bananas, parsley and spinach; zinc, a good source of which are carrots and ginger; and magnesium, which also occurs in the green foods.

Easy Does It	*Hi Mag*
Gingeroo	*Hit the Grass*
Ginger Spice	*Silky Strawberries*
Green Friend	*Sprout Special*

Urinary Infections
Cranberry juice is excellent for any sort of kidney and urinary infections. Cranberry is also thought to be good for an under-active thyroid, partly because it has traditionally been grown, particularly in the United States, in iodine-rich bogs. Cranberry juice on its own is much too strong for most people to handle. However, it mixes beautifully with any number of gentler juices like melon or apple. It will also add extra zest to basic vegetable juices like carrot. Cranberry is known for its cleansing properties, helping to rid not only the digestive system but other organs of the body of waste and bacteria. It is also said to be very good for skin problems such as acne.

Cranberry Cocktail

Water Retention
Water retention or oedema is a sign that the metabolism is not working properly and the body needs to be deep cleansed and rebalanced. It can be caused by many things, from hormones in birth control pills and Hormone Replacement Therapy, to hormone changes during the premenstruum and pregnancy. It can also be caused by food allergies and liver problems.

Encouraging the body to eliminate excess water from its tissues is a two-fold process. First, use natural diuretics such as nettle, dill, watermelon, grapes and cucumber that gently encourage the loss of excess water. Second, detoxify the system as a whole using the Juice Blitz. If swelling in the ankles is severe and prolonged it can indicate serious problems such as heart failure, so you need to check with your doctor. Check also for any possibility of food allergy if you have prolonged water retention, and decrease the amount of salt in your diet. The sodium/potassium balance in your body determines to a great extent whether the body eliminates excess fluids properly. Cut sugar from your diet.

Fight water retention by increasing the number of potassium-rich foods that you eat and make your juices from. These include: bananas, prunes, raisins, figs, seaweeds, fish, green vegetables, whole grains, kale, broccoli, spinach, Swiss chard, and all the other green foods, plus carrot and celery. You may be deficient in vitamin B6, which can interfere with the kidneys' ability to eliminate waste. Foods rich in B6 include molasses, brown rice, liver, eggs, cabbage and fish. Garlic, too, is one of the traditional foods for eliminating oedema from the tissues.

Black Watermelon *Green Zinger*
Cool as a Cuke *Potassium Power*
Dandelion Plus *Secret of the Sea*
Green Friend

Chapter Seven
Green Lightning

Once you get the basics of juicing under your belt – once you get used to the wild raw taste of fresh vegetables – you are ready for the next step: *green lightning*. And what a step it is. Green juices, like the foods they are pressed from, are little short of magical. They bring you increased energy, protection from radiation in the environment and from degenerative diseases as well as enhanced immune performance. Green foods help regenerate and rejuvenate the body. Go green and you can wave those annoying winter colds and 'flu good bye. The old adage 'eat your greens if you want to stay young and healthy' is now scientific fact. And the fun of it all is that, so far, advanced nutritional scientists know that green works wonders but nobody is yet sure why. The chlorophyll? The enzymes? Mystery ingredients? The very latest nutritional supplements have gone green – spirulina, chlorella, green barley, blue-green algae. The nutrients they contain – from vitamins and minerals to trace elements, enzymes and as yet unidentified health-promoting factors – are found there in perfect balance and synergy as well as in a highly bioavailable form. Your system just laps them up.

Bountiful Brassicas

Dark green vegetables such as broccoli, Brussels sprouts, collards, kale, kohlrabi and mustard greens have hit the headlines in the last few years thanks to an overwhelming abundance of medical and scientific evidence that they help prevent cancer. Prestigious North American medical journals such as the Journal of the National Cancer Institute and Federation Proceedings report that the sulphur and histidine in brassicas inhibit the growth of cancer tumours, detoxify the system of poisonous environmental chemicals, prevent colon cancer and increase the body's own supply of natural cancer-fighting compounds. They can also help lower low-density lipoproteins – the *bad* cholesterol – which accompany hardening of the arteries. They improve elimination and fight yeast infections too. Adding a couple of florets of broccoli or a few leaves of kale to a glass of carrot juice turns something good into something even better. But start slowly and gradually build up on the green. In the beginning – especially if you have a sweet tooth or if you are addicted to sugar – the taste can seem pretty strong. Build up gradually until you find that your old craving for sugars has actually been transformed into a new craving for green.

Grass That's Greener

Another group of green lightning foods, the cereal grasses, are some of the least known but most powerful green foods. You need special equipment to extract the juice from them, but these grasses are also sold in health food shops as a dried powder and can be stirred into raw juice by the teaspoonful. Of course grasses have been around for thousands of years, yet only in the last ten or fifteen years has the consumption of young grass – wheat or rye or oat or barley – begun to rise. In ancient times young cereal plants were treated with the respect they deserve. Tiny green tips of baby wheat plants were eaten as a delicacy in the Holy Land 2000 years ago. Then in the twenties and thirties, in the United States – before vitamin and mineral pills were in existence – bottled, dehydrated cereal grass became a popular food supplement.

Young grasses are very different from the mature grains they eventually turn into from which we make our breads and porridge. Dark green in colour, in some ways they are similar to dark green brassica vegetables in their protective abilities. But they are very special. When rice, wheat, corn, oats, barley, rye or millet are planted in good

GREEN LIGHTNING

healthy soil with plenty of rainfall and are harvested at
exactly the right moment not only do they taste sweet, but
are unbelievably rich in vitamins and minerals, enzymes
and growth hormones you would be hard pressed to find
elsewhere. They are *living foods* and the juice pressed from
them carries these life energies into your body. The young
germinated plant is a little miracle of nature. In the young
leaves photosynthesis produces simple sugars which are
transformed into proteins, fatty acids, nucleic acids such
as DNA and RNA as well as complex carbohydrates
through the action of enzymes and substrates produced
from minerals in the soil. The peak of nutritional bounty
in all cereal grasses – the moment when chlorophyll, protein and most of the vitamins and minerals reach their
zenith – occurs just before *jointing*. This is the moment at
which the young internodal tissue in the grass leaf starts to
elongate and form a stem. This is when cereal grasses are
best harvested – usually somewhere between 8 and 15 days
after planting. Afterwards the chlorophyll, protein and
vitamin content drops dramatically while the fibre content
increases rapidly. To give you some idea of just how
remarkable the nutritional content of young cereal grasses can be it is useful to compare fresh wheat grass to
freshly milled wholewheat flour:

Nutrients per 100 grammes dry weight:

	Wheat Grass	Wholewheat Flour
Chlorophyll (mg)	543	0
Vitamin A (iu)	23,136	0
Total Dietary Fibre (gm)	37	10
Protein (gm)	32	13
Carbohydrates (gm)	37	71
Calcium (mg)	277	41
Vitamin C	51	0
Iron	34	4
Folic Acid (mcg)	100	38
Niacin (mg)	6.1	4.3
Riboflavin (mg)	2.03	0.12

Green Blood

In 1928 the American chemist Charles Schnabel was searching for some material that could be added to poultry feeds to improve egg production and lower chicken mortality. He wanted what he described as a 'blood building material'. Scientists had discovered that chlorophyll – the green substance in plants – has a remarkable similarity in its chemical structure to haemo-globin – the oxygen-carrying element in animal blood. Schnabel figured that 'green leaves should be the best source of blood.' So he began to feed all sorts of green things to chickens – from alfalfa to combinations of twenty green vegetables. But he found them all wanting. Then he tried giving hens a green mixture which 'just happened to contain a large amount of immature wheat and oats.' Animals who got only 10 per cent of this cereal grass responded amazingly. Winter egg produc-tion shot up from an average of 38 per cent to 94 per cent of summer levels and the eggs that were produced had stronger shells and hatched healthier chicks.

Intrigued by his success with chickens, Schnabel began to investigate every aspect of cereal grasses – from the soils that produce the most nutritionally rich grasses to the effect that giving dehydrated grasses has on the health of humans. He also fed his own family of seven on them and was known to boast that none of them ever had a serious illness or a decayed tooth. He even developed a vision of how to feed the hungry of the world on the exceedingly high quality protein from cereal grasses.

The Grass Juice Factor

In the decades that followed other scientists working with animal nutrition confirmed that a mixture of young cereal grasses fed to livestock improved milk production in cows and produced stronger more resilient, longer-living animals – from guinea pigs and rats to rabbits, cats and ferrets. Others discovered that green cereal grass feeds, which are believed to contain natural plant steroid hormones, both enhanced fertility and improved lactation in many animals including humans. Since then scientists have done their best to isolate and identify the ingredient or ingredients in young cereal grasses responsible for all of this. Further research indicates that barley grass juice lowers serum cholesterol and that wheat grass, in addition to its rejuvenating powers, may have anti-cancer properties.

Those in the know have been making practical use of grasses for many years. Ann Wigmore, the founder of the Hippocrates Health Institute in Boston, has long promoted the use of wheat grass and wheat grass juice as well as green and raw foods in the treatment of chronic degenerative conditions.

Quantum Sunlight

Chlorophyll – the stuff that makes plants green – is an important health-promoting ingredient in young cereal grasses and green foods. The chlorophyll molecule has an ability to convert the energy of the sun into chemical energy through the mysterious process of photosynthesis. It is the chlorophyll molecule that enables plants to make carbohydrates out of carbon dioxide and water. All life on earth draws its power to be from the sun's energy, thanks to photosynthesis in plants.

Scientists now tend to believe that the remarkable health-promoting qualities of green plants reside in the synergistic effect of chlorophyll together with other vital nutrients, both known and unknown, that are found in the plants. H.E. Kirchner, who spent many years investigating the power of cereal grasses and green foods, has written, 'Chlorophyll, the healer, is at once powerful and bland – devastating to germs, yet gentle to wounded body tissues. Exactly how it works is still Nature's secret;

to the layman, at least, the phenomenon seems like green magic.' Little wonder that for thousands of years the leaves and green stems of plants have been used for supporting detoxification of the body, wound healing, deodorisation, and any number of other purposes.

Chlorophyll is known to inhibit the carcinogenic effects of exposure to simple environmental poisons such as coal dust and tobacco, and to foods such as red wine and fried beef. In fact chlorophyll used on its own for these purposes has been proved to be more effective than the anti-oxidant vitamins A, C and E. Simple chlorophyll also helps protect from radiation. And when two or more of the dark green vegetables and cereal grasses are used together an animal's resistance to radiation reaches a peak. Chlorophyll also inhibits the growth of bacteria by creating an environment in which they simply do not reproduce. It also decreases swelling and reduces inflammation and speeds wound healing while reducing itching, irritation and pain. The chlorophyll-rich green juices come into their own in the treatment of peptic ulcers and are also useful in the relief of a range of conditions including constipation, spastic colitis and halitosis.

Ask Any Weed

Some of the very best of the green foods to add to your raw energy juices are weeds – plants that grow wild in your garden or in fields and hedgerows in the country. Dandelions, nettles, ragweed and Lamb's Quarter are especially good sources of the minerals and trace elements that we tend to lack as a result of chemical farming. Nettles, for example, only grow on mineral-rich soils. A handful of young nettles (they don't sting yet) gives a great boost to a glass of carrot and apple juice. Dandelion, like nettle, is a natural diuretic – which is why in French its common name is *pissenlit* – and a blood cleanser and is stunningly rich in the carotenoids. Lamb's Quarter is not only rich in minerals but also tastes delicious and can be used in salads as well as juices without imparting too heavy a green flavour to whatever you are making. Comfrey, in small quantities, can be added to fresh juice. It is rich in allantoin which herbalists have long used to soothe intestinal irritations such as stomach ulcers and diarrhoea as well as to calm skin eruptions and heal wounds.

Seaweeds too are great additives to juicing. You can use powdered kelp, dried nori, arame, hiziki, laver bread, dulse, kombu and wakami or you can even slip a piece of fresh seaweed taken from unpolluted waters in the juicer next to your carrot. Seaweeds are full of trace elements which are essential to the body in minute quantities – elements such as boron, chromium, cobalt, calcium, iodine, magnesium, manganese, molybdenum, phosphorus, potassium, silicon and sulphur. Unlike the chalk which is added to bread to 'enrich' it with calcium, and most of the mineral supplements you buy in pill form in stores, the minerals in green plants such as these are *organic* which means that your body can easily make use of them to build health.

The Ultra Greens

Watercress and parsley are superb additions to your juices. They are ultra green and very powerful so you need very little to get a lot of benefit from them. Watercress contains many more organic minerals than spinach and is richer in vitamins too. It has a high sulphur content which experts in natural medicine claim helps to improve the functioning of the endocrine system. Thanks to its iron, manganese and copper content, it is also known to be good for strengthening the blood and relieving anaemia. And it is rich in vitamins C and E. Parsley is another natural diuretic – great for cleansing the body of wastes and reducing oedema. It is famous for its ability to improve the health of the kidneys and for its anti-oxidant compounds including beta-carotene. Like watercress juice, parsley juice is super-potent both in taste and in actions – you need only a stalk or two of either plant to turn any juice you are making into a green powerhouse.

Good, Better, Best

You can go green in three ways. Firstly, you can add a handful – a small one at first until you get used to green juicing – of kale or broccoli or dark green cabbage to a simple base such as half carrot and half apple. Secondly – and better still – you can grow organic cereal grasses like wheat grass or barley in trays and harvest as you need them (but you will need special equipment to juice them, as described in Resources, p. 147) to add to your vegetable juices. Finally, you can buy freeze-dried wheat grass or green barley or one of the other green magic foods such as spirulina or chlorella and add them to whatever juice you fancy.

Magic Spirals

Use the nutritious natural green additives freely. They will do you nothing but good. Queen of them all is spirulina. A near-microscopic, blue-green freshwater alga, spirulina is one of the finest green additives you will ever find. It is made up of translucent bubble-thin cells stacked end to end to form an incredibly beautiful green helix. $3^1/2$ billion years ago the blue-green algae began to fix nitrogen from the atmosphere and to convert it into carbon dioxide and sugars, releasing free oxygen in the process. This created the oxygen-rich atmosphere in which the rest of life was able to develop.

Spirulina is probably the single most important nutritional supplement you can use to support high-level health. It is unusual in that its protein is alkaline forming in the body rather than acid-forming. This can be very important for detoxifying the system and also for helping you deal with high levels of stress. Spirulina is also rich in vitamins E, B12, C, B1, B5 and B6 as well as beta-carotene, and the minerals zinc, copper, manganese and selenium. It also contains good levels of anti-ageing anti-oxidants and of *phycocyanin* – a blue pigment structurally similar to beta-carotene which experiments have shown can enhance immune functions. Finally, spirulina although very low in fat is rich in important essential fatty acids. Add between a teaspoon and a tablespoon to a glass of fresh juice, or mix a glass of fresh juice together with spirulina and a banana in a blender for a great breakfast drink.

Emerald Treasure

Chlorella, sometimes called the emerald food, is a green alga with pretty amazing properties, and it too is great as a juice additive. It gets its name from its high content of chlorophyll – the highest of any known plant. In addition it is rich in vitamins, minerals, fibre, nucleic acids, amino acids, enzymes, something called CGF – chlorella growth factor – and other important compounds. Chlorella is the biggest-selling health food supplement in Japan. Among the green foods, chlorella is known as the great normaliser, thanks to its apparent ability to alter bodily processes that are under- or over-active so that they return to normal. About 60 per cent of chlorella is protein. The vitamins it contains include vitamin C, beta-carotene and other carotinoids, thiamin, riboflavin, pyridoxine, niacin, pantothenic acid, folic acid, vitamin B12, biotin, choline, vitamin K, inositol and PABA. Chlorella is also rich in minerals and trace elements including phosphorus, potassium, magnesium, sulphur, iron, calcium, manganese, copper, zinc and cobalt.

Japanese scientists have discovered that chlorella can stimulate the production of white blood cells and enhance immunity as well as having anti-viral activity. It can also bind heavy metals such as cadmium, pesticide and herbicide poisons including PCB, and help remove them from the body. Meanwhile it helps protect the liver from toxic injury, and some practitioners claim it can help prevent hangovers by promoting the removal of alcohol from the body.

Easy Does It

The secret with using any of the green lightning foods – from crunchy broccoli to wheat grass or spirulina – is to start small and keep adding as you get used to the green. Generally speaking the worse your diet has been before you begin the less you will like the taste of the green foods at first. This is particularly true if you have always been a big sugar eater. Green lightning and sugar are at the opposite ends of the food continuum. This may be one of the reasons why going green with your juices is about the best thing you can do to counter low blood sugar, low energy problems or candida albicans. But once you get used to green you will love not only the way it makes you feel and look but even the way it tastes – so fresh and clean and alive.

Quantum Green Drink

Many green foods have strong plant structures and therefore can be difficult to break down in a juicer. That is why we prefer, when using watercress or parsley or one of the weeds, to pulverise them quickly in the blender by themselves before adding a freshly made glass of raw carrot, celery or apple juice and whisking the mixture together for a few seconds. This way you produce a therapeutic green drink that is equal to none. We have learned much from H.E. Kirchner, a world authority on the benefits of green foods. Here is our version of his famous 'Green Drink'. We call it Quantum Green.

Make a glass of carrot and apple juice or fresh pine-apple juice. Pour it into a blender and add a handful of sunflower seeds (which have been soaked in spring water overnight) as well as half the quantity of almonds and five dates without their stones. Now put in a handful or two of green leaves or sprouted green foods such as alfalfa or mung beans. Choose from comfrey, Lamb's Quarter, dandelion, parsley, mint, watercress, kale or beet top – using the leaves only, never the stems. Now liquefy the greens by blending for a few moments.

This is a rich protein food and an ideal meal replace-ment. If you want a less high-protein drink, leave out the seeds and nuts or cut their quantities in half.

Experiment with the green recipes on pages 118–119 and see what you come up with for yourself. Then let us know. We are always eager to find new ways of playing with green lightning.

Chapter Eight
Juice Freedom

We have examined the biochemical effect living juices have on the body. We have looked at the practicality of juicing and all the rites and rituals of deep cleansing and energising the body. But what can you expect from carrying out a Juice Blitz and then following the High Life Diet? What is it going to do for you? What are the real payoffs?

The Bottom Line

There are many, many rewards to be gleaned from the Juice High lifestyle. Your body gets healthier, energy soars, skin is clearer and less lined, eyes are brighter, weight problems lessen, and chronic depression or anxiety start to become things of the past. However, the truth is that when it comes to regular juicing and a Raw Energy lifestyle, nothing less than *freedom* is the bottom line. Incorporating the power of Raw Energy day after day into your life can not only bring freedom *from* negative experiences such as chronic fatigue and illness by strengthening immunity and deep cleansing of the body. It can also bring you freedom *to* do things – to be more creative and live out what you really are. Deep cleansing and regeneration help set people free. For we live in a difficult time, one which demands focused awareness and knowledge if we are to handle not only the physical toxicity in our environment but also the spiritual and emotional toxicity that distort our perceptions and limit the full expression of the unique soul energy which is within each one of us.

Only you can prove this for yourself by moving

beyond theory and getting into your own juicing programme. Then you can experience for yourself just how wonderful a personal revolution it can bring about.

Expand Your Horizons

When you detox your body you remove impediments to experience and to action. You release energy that has been suppressed beneath the physical burden of waste which we all carry. But the energy which is released needs to be channelled. While for most people the increase in energy which comes with a Juice High lifestyle grows gradually and steadily, for some it can be experienced as an explosion of life force which suddenly arises from within. This was Leslie's experience the first time she ever did a juice fast. This is her story:

'I had an important decision to make about my life, and I felt that I had neither the clarity nor the information I needed in order to be able to make it wisely. A doctor friend of mine who was an expert in detoxification suggested I try a fast. At first this sounded completely insane to me. What possible bearing could drinking juices and water have on decision making? Then he told me about all the ancient practices of using fasting for intellectual and spiritual ends. I learned how monks and nuns were fasted to clarify their inner vision and bring them spiritual awareness, how Pythagoras fasted for forty days and then insisted that his students fast also before sitting exams, and that the famous Swiss physician Paracelsus insisted that "Of all the remedies available, fasting is the greatest one." And I began to wonder.'

Gateway To Power

The Juice Blitz is but a milder form of detoxification than a fast on spring water. It will do the same thing but more slowly and more gently. And it is much easier on your system. It also has the advantage of not depleting your body of minerals and trace elements, as well as vitamins and other as yet unidentified metabolites which are central to high level health. The High Life Diet will continue the detoxification processes – yet more slowly and more gently still – while it carries through the metabolic building process to help restore first-rate biochemical functioning on which high-level health, emotional balance and mental and spiritual clarity depend.

'Still not entirely convinced, I began my juice fast which I continued for 21 days under medical super-vision. (This is the only way in which such a long juice fast should be carried out. More than two or three days on juice alone needs careful monitoring by a professional who understands and has experience with detoxification.) The results of my juicing quite literally changed my life. As a child and while I was growing up I had suffered endless illness – colds, flu, high fevers and nightmares every night. Then in my early twenties I found myself imprisoned by a heavy, long-term depression with no apparent cause for which no professional – doctor, psychologist or counsellor – could find a cure. Unknown to me it was juicing that would hold the key.

In the first five days on juice I experienced the odd headache and a great deal of fatigue since my body was throwing off waste at a fantastic rate. This temporarily depleted my energy for action so I rested as much as I could. Then the whole world began to look different. My body felt light instead of the burden I had for years experienced it to be. My eyes grew bright. But what amazed me most of all was that my whole experience of who I was began to shift. So did the way I viewed myself, my life, and the world around me.

Before my juice fast I had experienced myself as someone struggling against great odds day by day to just to raise my children and find my place in the world. During the detox I noticed that my image of myself and my attitudes towards life were undergoing subtle yet profound shifts. I began to see clearly and to feel that with steady commitment and patience I could accomplish what I wanted with my children and my work. I found that each day I would wake up free of the old anxieties, feeling fresh and excited about the day ahead.'

Wonderful Life

Someone once told Leslie a story about a psychologist who was studying the nature of optimism and pessimism in children. It's a story about just how different the world can look – depending on your attitude to life.

The psychologist filled a room with a tremendous array of toys of the kind that appeal to an eight-year-old – trains and trucks, building materials, stuffed toys, story books, painting and drawing materials. Then he took an eight-year-old *pessimist* and put him in the room while he and the child's mother waited in an adjoining office to see how long the child would amuse himself. In less than ten minutes the child came out of the room whining, 'Mummy, I'm bored. There's nothing to do in there.'

Next the psychologist replaced everything in the room with a large pile of horse manure. This time he sent an eight-year-old *optimist* into the room and closed the door, expecting that at any moment child would emerge. Instead, silence. Ten minutes passed. Then twenty. Finally an hour went by with no sign of the child. The child's mother voiced concern that perhaps her son had hurt himself. The psychologist let her open the door to see if her son was all right. Hearing the door open, the boy jumped up immediately and ran to his mother's arms shouting, 'Mummy, Mummy, there's a pony in here but I can't find him.'

Set Your Body Free

When it comes to physical strength and athletic prowess, juicing has real clout. After the Juice Blitz and ten days on the High Life Diet, your body becomes so much cleaner and clearer from inside out you no longer easily build up the wastes in the muscles and around joints that make exercisers and athletes so prone to injury. The kind of acidic buildup that comes with exercise is mini-mised, and you can work out longer and harder without pain. Replacing convenience foods with fresh foods and live juices also gradually stabilises blood sugar so that energy for physical activity is readily available and long-lasting. After three months of juicing a marathon fell runner described it this way: 'Everything has become effortless. I can run longer and harder without straining. Instead of demanding so much of my will, I find myself almost floating over the hills and rocks. Just occasionally it gets so good, I feel as though I could run on forever.'

Fuel for Change

We believe that the benefits of Juice High have the potential to be felt far beyond the individual. Social change is brought about by the dreams, the visions, the thoughts and the actions of people. The greater the clar-ity of perception and an individual's sense of freedom, the more creativity and potential benefit he or she can bring to work, relationships and society as a whole. Our educational system – despite the high-sounding phrases bandied around by ministers – is dedicated not to turn-ing out free-thinking, autonomous human beings but rather to 'normalizing' thought and behaviour. That way the status quo is maintained, and potent, active eccentrics whose visions go against the grain are kept in close check.

The goal of Juice High is diametrically opposed to this way of thinking. It is a potent tool for helping to establish freedom for each of us; the freedom to act according to our own perceptions and values and to pursue our own goals. These are goals which arise from the core of one's being rather than those which have been imposed from outside by parenting, schooling or the exploitative demands of our materialistic society.

Freedom is not, as advertisers would have us believe, drinking white rum on a tropical beach or wearing a pair of Levi 501s. Freedom is about living out the truth of your soul in the way you relate to others, in the work you do, in the creative pursuits and the choices you make. Of course such freedom is profoundly dangerous to those structures which would control us by delivering a pastiche of the real thing. Yet such freedom is the greatest high any of us ever experience – far better than any drug could offer. It is the freedom of learning to trust yourself.

Future Change

What is fascinating about real freedom is that it not only helps the individual experience and live out his or her own creativity, it also brings to our families, communities and the planet as a whole the very best that each of us has to offer.

Now, drinking a glass of green juice each morning and munching more carrots at lunch are not going to turn us into a Martin Luther King or a Mother Teresa. But they can go a long way towards helping us to clear away some of the physical, emotional and intellectual junk we have all picked up along the way that prevent us from being who we are, from seeing clearly, from trusting what we see and then acting on it. That is why we see *Juice High* as a practical, easy-to-use tool for personal transformation which can ultimately have a profoundly beneficial effect on the world around us. It is an exciting prospect.

Recipes

JUICE INDEX

There are several variables to be considered when formulating juice recipes. Fruit and vegetables have not yet been standard-ised (thank God) and vary considerably in size and juice yield. Not all centrifugal extractors are as efficient as others. Rather than give measurements in millilitres, we decided that the most practical way to present these recipes is by indicating roughly how many pieces of fruit and veg you'll need to make approxi-mately 280ml/10 fl. oz/half a pint. Also, Total Juices are made with a powerful blender rather than a centrifugal extractor.

Alfalfa – Father of all Juices

The word alfalfa means 'father of all grains' and when it comes to hair health you can't do better than alfalfa sprouts and carrot juice.

4–5 carrots   *Chopped parsley (optional)*
1 cup alfalfa sprouts

Juice as usual and top with some chopped parsley and drink.

Apples & Pears

Apples and pears are closely related and make a sublime com-bination when juiced together.

2 pears   *2 whole apples*

Juice as usual and drink straight away as this oxidises very quickly.

Apples, Celery & Fennel

2–3 apples   *1 bulb of fennel*
2 stalks celery

Apples, Pears & Berries

Berries are intensely-flavoured vitamin bombs that tend to be high in potassium and contain a remarkable range of other trace elements. Strawberries, raspberries, blackberries . . . in fact any berry works well when blended with apple juice, or apple and pear.

2 apples	*1 dozen berries (or as many as*
1 pear	*you like)*

Reserve a couple of pieces of apple to put through the juicer last and to flush the thick berry juice through the machine.

Apple Zinger

A terrific breakfast-time enlivener that perks up the whole system and really wakes up your taste buds.

2 or 3 whole apples	*1 (or more) 1cm cube of ginger*
1 whole lemon, peeled	

Atomic Lift-Off

This gives an immediate lift when you are feeling low. It's also a wonderful chaser for shots of tequila!

4–6 ripe tomatoes	*A pinch of cayenne pepper, or*
1 lime	*dash of Tabasco*

Juice the tomatoes and the lime (removing the skin but leaving the pith) then sprinkle with a dash of cayenne pepper.

Beetroot, Carrot & Orange

Beetroot enriches the blood and provides an excellent tonic for the kidneys. The sweetness of orange juice in this recipe will help you become accustomed to the earthy flavour of beet.

1 smallish beet	*1 orange*
4 carrots	

Save one of the carrots to put through the juicer last, as it will help to clear the machine.

Beet Treat

Profoundly powerful, this juice will give you sustained energy throughout the day.

$^1/_2$ whole beetroot (plus tops, if	*1 apple*
possible)	*1 stalk celery*
2 carrots	*3cm cucumber*

113

Black Watermelon

You have two choices on how to prepare this, you can juice the skin of the watermelon as well as the pink flesh and then add the molasses and stir in. Or, you can take only the pink flesh, put it into a blender or food processor, add the molasses and blend. We prefer the second method but either is good.

¹/₄ small watermelon   *1 tsp–1 tbsp blackstrap molasses*
                                              (unsulphured)

Carrot & Apple

This is the most basic juice cocktail; use it as the springboard for experimentation. Start by combining equal parts of the two juices and experiment until you find the proportions that suit you; we prefer one part apple to two parts carrot.

4 carrots   *1 apple*

Carrot & Orange

Peel the rind from oranges, but leave the pith, and put the whole fruit through the juicer together with the carrots.

1 orange   *4 carrots*

Carrot Milk

Adding soya milk to freshly-extracted carrot juice enhances its natural creaminess and gives you plenty of protein, without the clogging effect of cows' milk. Try adding the juice of a single small parsnip – scrubbed, topped and tailed but not peeled – and a little grated nutmeg.

3 carrots   *Soya milk to taste (or to fill the*
1 parsnip   *glass)*

Carrot Milk (Total Juice)

2 carrots   *Handful of ice cubes*
1¹/₂ cups soya milk   *Juice of ¹/₂ lemon*
    (see Resources, p. 147)   *Pinch of nutmeg*

Put carrots and soya milk into the blender with the ice cubes. Squeeze the lemon juice into the blender, blend for 30 seconds, top with fresh grated nutmeg and serve.

Carrot, Beet, Celery, Tomato

3 carrots	*2 stalks of celery*
1/2 beetroot, peeled	*2 tomatoes*

Carrot High

5 carrots	*1 clove garlic*
4 sticks celery	

Celery Sticks

3–4 sticks celery	*1 clove garlic*
4–5 carrots	

Juice as usual and drink immediately.

Chlorophyll Plus

A handful of dandelion leaves	*1 whole apple*
A handful of parsley	*A small bunch of grapes*
A handful of spinach	

Citrus Carrot Special

This is a beautiful drink made even better if you chill all of the ingredients before you use them.

2 carrots (juiced)	*1 small orange*
1/2 small pineapple	

Peel the orange and pineapple and cut into bite-sized pieces. Toss into the blender with a handful of ice cubes and the carrot juice. Blend and serve immediately.

Citrusucculent

1 ripe grapefruit (or pink grapefruit)	*1/2 ripe lemon*
	2 ripe oranges

Peel the fruit (leave the pith) and juice as usual.

Citrus Zinger

1 pink grapefruit	*1/2 lime*
1 orange	*1 (or more) 1cm cube of*
1/2 lemon	*ginger (optional)*

Cool as a Cuke

1 cucumber
1 clove garlic

1 tomato
dash of dill

Juice the vegetables and then sprinkle with ground dill and serve over ice.

Cranberry Cocktail

1 cup of cranberries
lemon juice

1 cup of sweet grapes or 2–3
apples

Put the grapes or cranberries and apples through the juicer then add a squeeze of fresh lemon juice before serving. If you don't have fresh cranberries you can use frozen ones.

Dandelion Plus

4–5 carrots
A handful of dandelion
leaves

1 bulb of fennel
lemon juice

Juice as usual then add a tablespoon of lemon juice to the mixture.

Double Whammy

4–5 carrots
A handful of dandelion
leaves

2 whole pears

Easy Does It

1 large green apple, whole
2 stalks celery

8–10 lettuce leaves

Juice as usual and drink before bedtime, or when you are feeling particularly tense.

Fab 5 Fruit Juice

A great fruit punch, this recipe can be varied and different fruits substituted according to seasonal availability.

½ apple
½ pear
1 tangerine, or similar

12 grapes
1 peach

116

Fatty Acid Frolic (Total Juice)

2 whole apples
2–3 dandelion leaves or
  large kale leaves or
  beetroot top

1 heaped tablespoon of fresh
  vacuum-packed linseeds
1 very ripe banana

Juice the apple and leaves as usual. Put into a blender with the linseeds and the banana and blend at high speed until smooth. Drink immediately.

Fruit Frappé (Total Juice)

This is a lovely drink rather like a frozen Daiquiri. Whether or not you add alcohol to it is up to you.

1/2 banana
1/2 orange, pith left on
1 mango, peeled, with the
  inner peel removed

1/2 cup of frozen strawberries
1/2 cup of soya milk or low-
  fat yoghurt
A handful of ice cubes

Cut the fruit into easy-to-manage pieces (obviously peel the banana and the orange), toss into the blender with the ice cubes and blend for 30 seconds at high speed. Serve immediately.

Fruit Medley (Total Juice)

1/4 small pineapple, peeled
  and cut into spears
1 small orange, peeled but
  with the pith left on

1/2 apple
1/2 banana
1 tbsp maple syrup or honey

Cut all the fruit into bite-sized pieces, place in the blender with a few ice cubes, turn on at high speed for half a minute. Serve immediately.

Ginger Berry

1 (or more) 1cm cube of
  fresh ginger
1 medium bunch of grapes

2 cups blackberries or
  raspberries

Juice as usual. You can also add some sparkling mineral water to this, or some ice; it makes a delicious and refreshing long drink on a hot day.

Gingeroo

Carrot and apple juice tastes even better if you ginger it up a little.

1 (or more) 1cm cube of
    fresh ginger

1 whole apple
4 carrots

Ginger's Best

¹/₂ cantaloupe melon
¹/₂ cm slice fresh ginger

1 lime (peel, leaving pith)

Ginger Spice

3 large carrots
1 whole pear

A small chunk of fresh ginger

Glorious Grapefruit

Apparently there is a world glut of pink grapefruits, which make a frothy, sweet and sharp juice that we love to drink for breakfast. Peel the fruit, but remember to leave as much of the white pith as possible to put through your juicer. Two grapefruits will yield slightly more than half a pint of juice.

Green Friend

3 whole apples
2–3 dandelion leaves or a
    couple of large kale leaves
    or beetroot top

A handful of mint

Green Goddess

This juice makes you smile like the *Mona Lisa*.

60ml (2 fl. oz) of carrot juice
60ml (2 fl. oz) of apple juice
60ml (2 fl. oz) of beetroot juice
60ml (2 fl. oz) of broccoli juice

¹/₂ tsp kelp powder
¹/₂ –1 tsp chopped fresh
    parsley
A squeeze of fresh lemon juice

Green Tomato

This invigorating green drink is not made with green tomatoes, which tend to be sour, but luscious red ones.

2–3 ripe tomatoes
2 stalks celery
1 green pepper

1/2 bulb of fennel
2–3 sprigs parsley/chopped
    parsley

Green Wild

2 whole green apples
2 stalks celery
1/4 lemon

1 (or more) 1cm cube of fresh
    ginger

Green Wow

2 green apples
4 stalks of celery

6 Chinese leaves
Juice of 10cm of cucumber

Green Zinger

2 kale leaves or beetroot tops
    or a handful of spinach

4–5 carrots
A small handful of parsley

Hi Mag

4–5 carrots
2 florets of broccoli

2 dandelion leaves, beetroot
    tops, spinach or kale leaves

Juice and season with a twist of lemon and a pinch of salt.

Hi NRG

1 apple
2 carrots

1 stalk of celery
Soya milk to taste

Hit the Grass (Total Juice)

A handful of fresh mint
A small pineapple, peeled
    and cut into convenient
    sized spears

A handful of any fresh cereal
    grass such as wheat or barley

Juice the mint and pineapple in your ordinary juicer, then juice the cereal grass in a wheat-grass juicer. Whisk together. Alternatively, pour the fruit juice into a food processor or blender and toss the cereal grasses in, blend with the blade until highly blended, then pour through a strainer to remove the indigestible fibre. Serve over ice. This can also be made using a teaspoon to a tablespoon of any of the freeze-dried cereal grasses such as barley grass or wheat grass.

Lazy Lettuce

2 whole apples   *5 lettuce leaves*

Lemon Zinger

1 whole apple   *Sparkling mineral water*
¹/₂ a lemon

Juice the apple and the lemon – leaving the white pith on the lemon – pour into a glass and top up with sparkling water and ice.

Leslie's Cocktail

Bananas are not totally unjuiceable if you use very ripe fruit. Put them through your juicer first, then the apples, which will help to flush the thick banana through the machine. Alternatively, use a blender to make the breakfast of champions. This recipe also works well with melon in place of apple.

180ml (6 fl. oz) of fresh apple   *1 tsp each of spirulina, chlorella,*
*   juice*   *   and green barley powder*
1 ripe banana

Linusit Perfect

This recipe is replete with valuable essential fatty acids – both omega-6 and omega-3 – which are often deficient in people who have been surviving on the typical Western fare of convenience foods. It must be made with freshly ground vacuum-packed linseeds or flaxseeds for these precious fatty acids are highly unstable and go rancid quickly.

2 whole apples   *3 carrots*
¹/₂cm slice of ginger   *1 tbsp linseeds or flaxseeds*

Juice the fruit, carrots and ginger as usual. Place the linseed in a coffee grinder and grind finely. Then add to the glass of juice, stir well and drink immediately. Alternatively you can put the linseed into a food processor, grind and then pour the freshly made juice in and blend for 3 seconds.

Merry Belon

Berries are one kind of fruit that combines really well with melons and the array of flavours gives lots of scope for experimentation. Try galia & raspberry, honeydew & blackberry or the classic watermelon & strawberry.

1 slice of watermelon, 3cm wide and cut into chunks to fit your juicer

6 strawberries, washed and with their green stalks removed

In hot weather, a good tip is to freeze the berries before juicing them.

More Raw NRG

Like the Raw NRG cocktail, More Raw is based on the crucial combination of carrot and apple, with green vegetable juices diluted by cucumber and celery. When making this juice, put the ingredients through your juicer in reverse order and you'll end up with a greenish drink tinged with orange froth.

3 carrots
1 apple
2 stalks of celery
3cm section of cucumber

1 broccoli floret
A small bunch of spinach or watercress (or dandelion leaves)

Orange Tonic

2 oranges
1 (or more) 1cm cube of fresh ginger

Sparkling water

Juice the ginger and orange as usual, pour into a glass and top up with sparkling mineral water. This is particularly delicious in winter.

Papaya & Pineapple

This exotic combination is especially good for settling upset stomachs.

½ small pineapple, cut into spears

1 mango

Take care to remove all the flesh from the stone of the mango before you juice it.

Parsley Passion

Another vegetable rich in mineral salts is parsley. Drinking parsley juice daily can bring relief to people troubled by allergies.

1 bunch parsley   *2 apples*
3–5 carrots   *2 small cauliflower florets*

Parsnip Perfect

Parsnips, also know as anaemic carrots, are well known for their ability to strengthen hair, skin and nails and can protect against hair loss.

2 parsnips   *1 beetroot*
3 carrots

Pepper Upper

This juice is a great replacement for tea breaks and mid-afternoon pick-me-ups of coffee and biscuits. It helps you to sizzle with vitality without any of the downside you get from sugar and caffeine.

2 carrots   *¼ bunch of watercress*
1 red pepper   *2–3 sprigs of parsley*
1 stick celery

Save one of the carrots until last to clear out any juice left inside your machine. Otherwise, put the ingredients through in any order, stir and serve.

Pineamint

Especially good if taken at bedtime for settling the stomach and helping you sleep.

1 small pineapple   *A small bunch of fresh mint*
                                    leaves

Remove the skin of the pineapple and cut into convenient spears. Juice as usual and serve over ice for a long summer drink.

Pineappage

This may seem like a weird combination, but it's one way to sweeten the mega-nutrient fix of fresh cabbage.

1/4 large pineapple cut into spears   *1/3 green cabbage*

Pineapple Grapefruit Drink

1 small pineapple   *1 peeled grapefruit*

Pineapple Green

To 180ml (6 fl. oz) of freshly extracted pineapple juice add one or more of the following:

1 tsp–1 tbsp of powdered wheat grass, green barley, spirulina or chlorella

Popeye Punch

1 whole apple – including seeds   *A small handful of spinach*
4 or 5 carrots   *1 cucumber*

Potassium Power (Total Juice)

1 yellow or green melon, such as cantaloupe, honeydew etc.   *A pinch of grated nutmeg*
6 cubes ice (made with spring water)
1 over-ripe banana

Scoop out the flesh of the melon, place in a food processor or blender, add the banana, blend well, pour into a glass over the ice cubes and sprinkle with a pinch of freshly ground nutmeg.

Potassium Punch

Our tribute to N.W.Walker, the American raw food pioneer and evangelist of detoxification; drink it religiously!

3 carrots   *A few stalks of fresh coriander or parsley*
2 stalks celery
4–6 leaves of lettuce or winter greens   *A handful of spinach or watercress (or dandelion leaves)*

Pulp Gazpacho (Total Juice)

You can also make wonderful raw soups as well as uncooked warm soups using total juicing methods.

2 cups of spring water
1 medium sized carrot
1 stick celery
2 spring onions
4 ripe tomatoes, chilled

1 tsp Marigold Swiss vegetable
   bouillon powder (see
   Resources, p. 147)
A dash of white wine
1 tsp parsley

Place all the ingredients in the blender. Add two or three ice cubes, blend for 30 seconds, sprinkle with parsley and serve.

Quantum Green (Total Juice)

A super-charged blender drink enriched with sprouted pulses and sunflower seeds. Apples can be substituted for the pineapple.

3 carrots
2 spears of pineapple
1/4 cup soaked sunflower seeds

1/4 cup assorted sprouts
A handful of spinach leaves.

Juice the spinach with the carrots, then cut the pineapple into chunks and put into the blender with the sprouts and seeds. Blend together, adding the freshly made juice.

Raw NRG

Carrot and apple juice is the basis for this health-packed cocktail, which is devised to promote all-round health with the addition of celery and cucumber to the carrot and apple base. As you become more adventurous in your juicing, try reducing the apple content and adding green leaves of cabbage, spinach or dandelion to increase the green energy content.

1 apple
4 carrots
1 or 2 stalks of celery

5 cm section of cucumber
1 cm cube of fresh ginger
   (optional)

The addition of a cube or two of ginger gives the Raw NRG mix a real zing.

Red Cool

The addition of a cube or more of ginger makes Red Cool red hot.

1 beetroot   1 (or more) 1cm cube of fresh
2 apples   ginger
4 carrots

Red Devil

This recipe provides a real tonic for the blood and is a great
source of vitamins A, B-complex, C, D, beta-carotene, vitamins
K and E as well as calcium, iron, potassium, magnesium,
manganese, sulphur, iodine and copper. It's also useful for
clearing infections of the urinary tract and upset stomachs.

3 carrots   1 beetroot
3 stalks celery

Put the carrots and celery in the juicer first and then add the
beetroot. If feeling extravagant, serve with half a teaspoon of
fresh cream floated on the top.

Red Flag

3 small ripe tomatoes   A handful of spinach
4 carrots

Red Genius

4 carrots   3cm section of cucumber
1 large raw beetroot

Rhubarb Radiance

Drink at night before bed.

2 large stalks rhubarb   3 medium apples

Roots Soup

Root vegetables are the best source of B-complex vitamins.
Here, their thick, sweet and creamy juices are complemented
by the aniseed flavour of fennel. Dilute your roots soup with
cucumber juice, but if it's still too thick add a splash of spring
water.

1/2 smallish beetroot   1/2 bulb of fennel
1 medium-sized parsnip   5cm section of cucumber
1 sweet potato

125

Salad Juice

4–5 carrots   3–4 radishes
4 sticks celery

Salsa Surprise

2 large ripe tomatoes   A small bunch of parsley
3 carrots   1 clove garlic
2 sticks celery

Scary Mary

See Virgin Mary

Secret of the Sea (Total Juice)

4 carrots   2 sheets nori seaweed
2 whole apples

Juice the apple and carrot then pour into a blender along with the seaweed. Blend thoroughly and serve. This is even better if you toast the seaweed under a grill or near a flame or hotplate, very briefly – it takes no more than 10 or 15 seconds to do on both sides. You can then break it up into the juice and blend.

Silky Strawberries (Total Juice)

Strawberries are surprisingly potent when it comes to support-ing a body that is under stress. Just 100gms of strawberries contain as much as 80mg vitamin C, as well as all the other vitamins except for B12 and D, plus valuable minerals. Strawberries have a natural diuretic action and are very calming to the liver. They also contain salicylic acid which, according to experts in natural medicine, is good for any sort of kidney or joint complaint.

2 cups strawberries   1 ripe banana
1 ripe pear   A handful of fresh mint leaves

Juice the strawberries and pear as usual then place in a blender with the banana and mint and blend until smooth. This drink is particularly delicious when made with a frozen banana; it takes on the taste and consistency of a natural ice-cream.

Smooth as Silk (Total Juice)

This recipe is rich in natural fruit sugars, potassium, magnesium and the amino acid tryptophan which can be turned into serotonin in the brain. It is also absolutely irresistible.

2 cups blackberries, either   *1 whole banana*
   fresh or frozen
1 ripe apple

Juice the berries and the apple. Put the juice and banana into a food processor or blender and blend until smooth. Drink 45 minutes before bedtime.

Spicy Apple

2 apples, whole   *A pinch of cinnamon*
1 lime

Juice the apples and the lime (leave the pith on the lime), sprinkle with cinnamon and serve.

Spicy Carrot

This juice is a great source of minerals such as magnesium, potassium, calcium, iron, sulphur, copper, phosphorus and iodine, as well as anti-oxidants, beta-carotene, vitamins A, C, E and niacin, vitamins D and K. It will also soothe a slightly delicate stomach. Braeburn and Cox's are ideal for this juice, but any sweet apple will do.

4 carrots   *A pinch of ground cinnamon*
2 spears of pineapple   *A pinch of ground nutmeg*
1 Braeburn or Cox's apple

Pineapples vary considerably in size. You'll need half a small one or a quarter of a big one. Remove the fibrous skin with a sharp knife and cut into long spears that will fit into your juicer. The cinnamon and nutmeg can be sprinkled on top of the freshly-extracted juice, or stirred into it as you prefer.

Spiked Celery

4 stalks celery   *1 clove garlic*
4–5 carrots

JUICE HIGH

Spinapple

When you mix apple with spinach you have an amazing combination for cleansing the digestive tract and improving elimination quickly, probably because spinach (which is high in oxalic acid) combines with the pectin in the apple's mineral salts to form a unique compound that has remarkable cleansing actions. Some practitioners in natural medicine claim that it actually clears old encrusted faeces that has accumulated over months and years in the colon making it possible to eliminate it from the body.

3 whole apples   *A handful of spinach*

Drink twice a day; especially important just before bedtime.

Spring Salad

3 florets of broccoli   *1 clove of garlic*
4 carrots   *1 tomato*
2 stalks of celery

Sprouting o' the Green

2 cups of alfalfa sprouts   *A few sprigs of parsley*
2 cups of mung bean sprouts   *2 apples*
1 carrot

Sprout Special

This juice is rich in natural phyto-hormones that help protect the body from the damage that petrochemically derived pesticides and herbicides can foster. It is also enormously rich in life-enhancing enzymes.

4 carrots   *1 cup sprouted seeds (mung*
1 whole apple   *beans, alfalfa, chickpeas,*
                                    adzuki beans, etc)

Sprinkle some grated ginger on top or a little cinnamon and serve over ice.

Straight CJ

When buying carrots, choose those with the darkest colour. Size doesn't matter, but many of the recipes in this book refer to 'medium-sized' carrots, around 15cm in length. Whichever variety you use, you'll need about a pound, or half a kilo of carrots to make 280ml or 10fl.oz juice. As a rule of thumb, we reckon that half a dozen medium carrots will yield about half a pint of juice. Scrub them under cold running water and remove the tops and tails, but it is not necessary to peel carrots before putting them through the juicer.

Sweet and Spicy

2 whole apples
2 x 1cm cube fresh ginger

½ small pineapple cut into
  convenient-sized spears

Juice as usual, adding as much ginger as you like, and sprinkle with a little ground cinnamon.

Sweet Salvation

Sweet capsicums (peppers) contain more vitamin C than oranges. Here, the juice is blended with freshly-made tomato juice to produce a deep red-orange, sweet yet savoury drink.

1 red or yellow pepper
2 ripe tomatoes (or 1 beef
  tomato)

1–2 carrots
3cm section of cucumber

Tomato & Carrot, Celery & Lime

A deliciously light combination (and not a bad medium for pepper vodka):

2–3 ripe tomatoes
2 carrots

2 stalks of celery
½ lime

Top of the Beet

1 apple
5 carrots

3 leaves of beetroot top
A handful of parsley

Tossled Carrot

5 big carrots
1 whole apple

A pinch of turmeric

Juice the carrots and apple, pour into glasses and sprinkle with turmeric.

Tropical Prune

*1 small pineapple, peeled
and cut into
convenient-sized
spears*

*2 fresh prunes – when prunes
are not in season, substitute
one pear*

Juice as normal, then grate a pinch of nutmeg on to the top and serve.

Vegetarian

*4 carrots
1/2 bulb of fennel
1 apple
1 lime*

*Either a handful of fresh
cereal grass or 1 tsp–1 tbsp
powdered green
supplements*

Juice all ingredients except for the cereal grasses, then put the juice and the cereal grasses in a blender or food processor and blend thoroughly. Strain before serving to remove the indigestible fibre. If you use a powdered green supplement as well, then juice as normal, pour the juice into the food processor or blender, add the powdered green supplement, blend and serve over ice.

Vampire Mary

See Virgin Mary, below.

Virgin Mary

A Bloody Mary without the vodka, we find that the flavour of this refreshing tomato-based cocktail benefits from a few drops of Tabasco. Add a clove of garlic and it becomes a Vampire Mary; a fresh jalapeno or other hot green chilli pepper turns it into a Scary Mary.

*2 ripe tomatoes
2 carrots
1/2 beetroot*

*1 stalk celery
1 cucumber*

Waterfall

*5cm section of cucumber
1 whole apple*

*3 carrots
1/2 smallish beetroot*

HIGH LIFE RECIPES: SALADS

Trio Salads

Trio Salads are best of all. The principles of making them are simple. Mix together three vegetables – one root, one bulb (or 'fruit') vegetable, and one leaf vegetable. Garnish with fresh or dried herbs and add dressing.

Root vegetables: carrots, celeriac, turnips, onions, leeks, beetroot, radishes, white radishes, etc.

Bulb or 'fruit' vegetables: tomatoes, red and green peppers, fennel, avocado, cucumber, cauliflower, celery, broccoli, courgettes, mushrooms, calabrese, etc.

Leaf vegetables: lettuce, young dandelion leaves, young beet tops, red or white cabbage, Brussels sprouts, spring onions, spring greens, spinach, chicory, endive, etc. Watercress, cress and sprouted grains and seeds can be used in any combination, or on their own, or as a garnish.

To increase a salad's protein content you can sprinkle it with three-seed mixture, an excellent source of both omega-3 and omega-6 essential fatty acids. Mix together equal quantities of sunflower, pumpkin and sesame seeds, grind in a coffee grinder, then sprinkle on the salad. Three-seed mixture can also be added to breakfasts and to drinks. Once ground it should be stored in the refrigerator. You can also give salads a protein lift with mixed nuts, or sprouted seeds or grains, or add some soft goat's cheese, free-range chicken, chopped boiled eggs, prawns, etc.

Sprout Salad

Mix two or three kinds of sprouted grains or seeds (a handful of each) in a bowl, add half a sliced avocado and season with fresh basil and chives. Garnish with black olives and dress with garlic dressing.

Spinach Splendour

2 cups spinach   *1 cup fresh mushrooms*

Remove stems and veins of spinach. Slice mushrooms finely and mix together. Toss in garlic dressing and sprinkle with basil or sunflower seeds.

131

Red Slaw

1¹/2 cups grated cabbage
1 grated carrot
¹/2 grated green pepper

1 tbsp honey
A pinch of celery seeds

Toss with salad dressing and serve.

Sunshine Salad

The fresh pineapple gives this salad a tropical taste. Make sure your pineapple is ripe by pulling out one of its centre leaves; if it comes out easily it is ready to eat.

A few crisp lettuce leaves
1 fresh pineapple
2 carrots
2 sticks celery
¹/2 green pepper

2 handfuls of sultanas (or raisins)
¹/2 tsp celery seeds
1 tsp dry mustard mixed with vinaigrette

Wash and crisp the lettuce leaves in the fridge. Peel the pineapple (it is not necessary to core it) and cut it into fairly small cubes. Coarsely grate the carrots, and finely chop the celery and green pepper, and add them to the pineapple cubes. Add the sultanas, soaked in water for a few hours to plump them up. Sprinkle with celery seeds and serve on a bed of crisp lettuce leaves. Serve with a piquant mustardy mayonnaise or French dressing.

Orange Orange Salad

A surprising combination . . . but it works!

4 carrots
6 oranges
1–2 cups white cabbage

2 handfuls of raisins or small seedless grapes
4 tsp sesame seeds

Coarsely chop the carrots. Juice four of the oranges and blend the juice with the carrots until you have a smooth mixture. Finely shred or grate the cabbage and put it in a bowl with the raisins or grapes. Pour the carrot mixture over it and lightly mix with a fork. Sprinkle with the sesame seeds and garnish with the two remaining oranges, peeled and sliced.

Summer Symphony

This salad is an exciting play of colours and shapes – the more variety the better.

1 lettuce (cos is good)	6 cherry tomatoes
1 cup small cauliflower florets	4 radishes (sliced)
2 celery stalks (finely chopped)	1 green pepper (cut into thin strips)
	Watercress
2 carrots (finely grated or cut into matchsticks)	Fresh sweetcorn or alfalfa sprouts to garnish

Place the lettuce leaves, torn into bite-sized pieces or shredded, into a bowl – a clear glass bowl is nice for this one so that all the beautiful colours show through it. Prepare the vegetables and arrange in layers in the bowl, keeping the watercress for decoration. Dress with a thinned mayonnaise dressing, perhaps blended with a tomato or two, and top with sweet corn or alfalfa sprouts, and sprigs of watercress.

Sprout Magic Salad

Make a base with alfalfa or mung sprouts and around the dish arrange:

grated carrot	sliced mushrooms
red cabbage	black olives
white cabbage	spring onions
beetroot	

Sprinkle raisins over the grated vegetables and spoon over a rich dressing.

SALAD DRESSINGS

Basic Dressing

Mix one part lemon juice and two parts extra virgin olive oil or four parts mashed avocado. Add herbs, garlic, mustard or honey to this base.

Tomato Dressing

3–5 tomatoes	1/2 tsp basil
2 tbsp lemon juice	

Put into a blender and liquefy. Store in the fridge.

133

Avocado-Tomato Dressing

4 small tomatoes
1 avocado
2 tbsp lemon juice

A dash of Tabasco
1 crushed clove of garlic or
   a dash of garlic powder

Mix in a blender. Store in the fridge.

Yoghurt and Egg Dressing

1 egg yolk
1¹/2 cups non-fat yoghurt
   or tofu
3 tbsp lemon juice or cider
   vinegar

A pinch of cayenne pepper
Fresh or dried herbs to taste
2 tsp honey

Put the ingredients into the top of a double boiler and stir over hot water until the mixture thickens. Refrigerate to serve cold or use hot, on hot potato salad or hot rice salad.

Thousand Island Dressing

1 hard-boiled egg, chopped
5 tsp celery, finely chopped
3 tbsp onion, finely chopped
2 tbsp black olives, chopped

1 tbsp green pepper, finely
   chopped
¹/2 cup non-fat yoghurt

Mix all the ingredients together and serve chilled.

Non-Oil Vinaigrette

3 tbsp dried skimmed milk
¹/2 tsp Dijon mustard
2 tsp honey
A dash of pepper

A pinch of basil
1 clove garlic, crushed
2 tbsp vinegar

Mix the ingredients, adding the vinegar last. Beat well or blend until smooth. Chill and use the same day.

RAW SOUPS

Cucumber

1 cup low fat yoghurt or
   soya milk
¹/2 cucumber, peeled and
   sliced

A sprig of mint
1 tsp lemon juice

Blend and serve sprinkled with parsley.

Gazpacho (see also Pulp Gazpacho, p. 124)

4–6 peeled tomatoes	2 sticks of celery
3 carrots	A dash of cayenne

Put through a juicer, sprinkle with chopped chives and diced green pepper.

Avocado Smoothie

³/4 cup low-fat yoghurt or tofu	1 tsp lemon juice
¹/2 avocado	1 chopped spring onion
¹/4 diced red pepper	A dash of Tabasco

Blend and serve.

Carrot Chowder

1 cup nuts (almonds, hazels or pecans)	2 tsp vegetable bouillon powder (see Resources, page 147)
1 cup low-fat yoghurt	3 cups carrot juice (using about 12 big carrots)
2 egg yolks	Ice cubes
1 tbsp olive oil	¹/2 green pepper
Small clove of garlic	2 spring onions
Juice of ¹/2 lemon	Chopped parsley

Grind the nuts finely and blend them with the yoghurt, egg yolks, pressed garlic, lemon juice, olive oil and seasoning. Juice the carrots into a jar with ice cubes in it, then slowly add the juice and ice to the yoghurt mixture, stirring well. Serve sprinkled with a mixture of finely chopped green pepper, spring onion and parsley.

Flamingo Soup

2 medium-sized beetroot	1 tbsp fresh thyme
10 carrots	1 tbsp fresh basil
1 small head celery	Marigold Swiss vegetable bouillon powder (see p. 147) to taste
Ice	
Juice of 1 lemon	
4–6 tomatoes	6 tbsp yoghurt
2 handfuls almonds	Chives

Juice the beetroot, carrots and celery and put into an airtight jar with some ice and the lemon juice. Blend the tomatoes, almonds, thyme, basil and bouillon powder. Combine the two mixtures and serve in bowls with a spoonful of yoghurt and a sprinkling of chopped chives.

Fresh Green Soup

2 avocados, peeled and
    stoned
3 cups apple juice
Juice of ½ lemon
1 courgette
A handful of alfalfa and
    mung sprouts
1 stick celery

Parsley
2 tsp tamari
1 tsp Marigold Swiss vegetable
    bouillon powder (see
    Resources, p. 147)
Ground ginger
Sliced mushrooms or flaked
    almonds

Combine the avocados, apple juice, lemon juice, parsley, tamari, vegetable bouillon and a pinch of ginger in the blender. Grate the courgette and finely dice the celery and mix them with the sprouts. Now pour on the avocado sauce. Serve sprinkled with sliced mushroom or flakes of almond.

MUESLI

Live Muesli

1–2 tbsp breakfast oats,
    soaked overnight in a
    little spring water

1 grated apple (or mango,
    peach, strawberries, etc)
½ cup low fat yoghurt

Mix all the ingredients and sprinkle with toasted seeds or mixed nuts.

PARTY TIME

Raw juices are seriously good for you. But who wants to be serious all the time? Not only is it OK to have fun, but making time to relax and enjoy yourself is crucial. Raw juices are not just for the abstemious and self-consciously healthy; they're also utterly delicious and appeal to the hedonist inside all of us.

Naturally sweet, fruity drinks are the healthy alternative to sugary pop that usually fuels children's parties and tends to make kids hyperactive, not to say stroppy. We can't guarantee that your child's birthday party won't end in tears if you give the young guests raw juice instead of fizzy drinks and fruit smoothies instead of ice cream sundaes, but our experience suggests that children will get a lot less fractious and play more happily together if you do.

Not that there is anything childish about the kind of fruit punches suggested in this section. Mixed with alcohol, freshly extracted juices make the most seductive cocktails and are guaranteed to make any social gathering flow easily. Which is not to suggest that getting intoxicated on a regular basis is a great idea, but that the expansive conviviality induced by alcohol helps us all to remember that we're only human.

Raw juices make the most sublime mixers for alcohol, but at any adult gathering there will be a proportion of people who do not wish to drink alcohol. Raw juice is a great leveller at parties because you can devise cocktails that taste just as good with or without a shot of alcohol. Teetotallers and hard-core hedonists can then mingle with impunity, all cradling glasses that look the same.

The first time we observed this phenomenon was at a marathon poetry performance for which we concocted a Purple Poetry Potion. It being an evening of beat poetry reading we used beetroot juice, mixed with apple and pear, with or without vodka. Beat poets have varying needs. Some wanted a stiff drink to steady their nerves; others were in rehab and scrupulously avoided stiff drinks. All, however, were intrigued by the profoundly earthy potion and some were moved to new heights of lyricism!

SMOOTHIES

Children of all ages love smoothies, made in a blender rather than a juicer, which is particularly appropriate for liquefying bananas. Bananas *are* juiceable if you use very soft specimens and follow them through your juicer with very watery fruits such as melons, which will help to wash the thick banana through the machine. However, using a blender to make banana drinks is a lot easier and less wasteful.

Many soft exotic fruits including peaches and mangoes, papaya and pineapple work well in the blender (so long as you take care to remove all their skin and stones). Smoothies are especially good when blended with plain yoghurt, which give them the texture of milk shakes, or melted ice cream with a low fat content. Use low-fat yoghurt, or Greek yoghurt made with goats' milk. These are a few of our favourite combinations:

Banana & Pineapple Smoothie

1 banana   *3 tbsp low-fat yoghurt*
2 spears of pineapple

Peel the banana and break into chunks. Remove the fibrous skin from the pineapple and cut into spears, then into chunks. Put all the ingredients into the blender and blend until smooth.

Mango & Peach Smoothie

If you have a problem getting the stone out of a mango, the trick is to use a tablespoon. Cut around the edge of the fruit with a sharp knife. Slide the spoon over one side of the stone and twist it.

1 mango   *3 tbsp low-fat yoghurt*
3 peaches

Stone the mango and the peaches and cut both fruits into chunks. Put all the ingredients into the blender and blend until smooth.

Banana & Peach Smoothie with Strawberries

1 banana   *12 strawberries*
1 peach   *3 tbsp low-fat yoghurt*

138

Peel the banana and break it up into chunks. Remove the stone from the peach and chop it into chunks. Remove the green stalks from the strawberries. Put all the ingredients into the blender and blend until smooth.

Cantaloupe & Papaya Smoothie   *V. G.*

Cantaloupe melons, with their rough skins and flesh of a delicate pink, orange or green colour, produce a rich, sweet juice that blends well with other exotic fruits.

½ cantaloupe melon   *1 papaya* */ mango*

Cut the melon into spears, remove the flesh from the skin. Peel the papaya and scrape out the seeds. Chop both into chunks, put into the blender and blend until smooth. You can use mango instead of papaya and you may also like to add a piece of citrus fruit – an orange, or maybe a lime – to add another dimension.

Banana & Honeydew with Apricot   *V. G.*

A mild, quite thick nectar that is best served over ice, or thinned with a splash of spring water. Less than half a honeydew should be more than adequate. Cut the melon into spears, then slice the flesh into chunks and remove from the skin.

1 banana   *6 apricots*
⅓ honeydew melon

Peel the banana, stone the apricots and remove the flesh from the melon. Put all the ingredients into a blender and blend until smooth.

EXOTIC FRUIT COCKTAILS

International commerce has blurred the seasons so that there is an abundant supply of exotic fruits in the supermarkets all year round, but summer is the right time to make the most of them. Exotic fruity cocktails made with a centrifugal juice extractor have an amazingly creamy texture and are perfect refreshment for a hot afternoon. For garden parties and barbecues, they're ideal.

The recipe suggestions below could be enlivened with the addition of a jigger of rum, or maybe a splash of vodka: far be it for us to discourage experimentation. The ideal way to chill these drinks is with a handful of crushed ice in the bottom of each glass, but it's also a good idea to keep all the ingredients refrigerated or iced in an insulated box.

Melon Medley with Berries

You can mix different kinds of melon juice together to create sublime blends, such as Honeyloupe (cantaloupe and honeydew, which is even better with a hint of ginger). Add summer berries to perk up their flavour. Use this recipe as the basis for experimentation.

1 slice watermelon   *12 raspberries*
1 slice honeydew

Peel the waxy outer skin from the honeydew and wash the rind of the watermelon. Juice the ingredients together and serve over ice.

Cantaloupe and Carrot with a Twist of Lemon

An intriguing and refreshing combination with a marvellous colour.

1/2 cantaloupe melon   *1/2 lemon*
3 carrots

Remove the rind from the melon with a vegetable peeler and the skin from the lemon, leaving the pith. Juice together, leaving one of the carrots to put through your juicer last.

Kiwi and Grape with Honeydew

Kiwis do not have to be peeled before juicing, so long as they're thoroughly washed. They have a slightly sharp flavour that blends well with melon and this juice is light, green and refreshing.

2 kiwi fruits   *12 green grapes*
1/4 honeydew melon

Peel the waxy rind from the melon and put the flesh through the juicer with the other ingredients.

Orangeade

Forget about proprietary canned drinks and make your own sparkling summer cooler.

2 oranges	*¹/₄ lime*
¹/₄ lemon	*Soda or sparkling spring water*

Peel the citrus fruits, leaving on the white pith, and serve, topping up the glass with soda or sparkling water.

Orange & Raspberry

A terrific, summery combination with an amazing colour.

2 oranges	*A handful of raspberries (about 12)*

Peel the oranges, leaving on the pith, and juice as usual with the raspberries.

Pinorange

Pineapple and orange is a great, refreshing combination. Oranges vary considerably in juiciness: you'll need one big, firm, luscious orange or two smaller specimens.

2 spears of pineapple (about ¹/₂ a smallish fruit)	*1 or 2 oranges*

Peel the fibrous outer skin from the pineapple and the waxy skin from the orange, leaving the pith. Juice together.

THE ALCOHOL CONNECTION

The juices used in most cocktail bars come out of a carton and are rarely fresh, but you can set up a raw juice bar to make drinks that taste superb and are nourishing as well as intoxicating! Raw juice is especially useful for mixing with the clear spirits, particularly vodka, but be careful how much you add, since raw juice cocktails are deceptively easy to drink. Remember the golden rule of moderation in all things.

Cocktails were originally invented during Prohibition in America to disguise the harsh taste of illegally-distilled hooch. However, we never touch cheap liquor and recommend that you stick to the more refined premium brands, which have been distilled to a higher specification and will leave you with less of a hangover.

The exception to the quality rule is when mixing juices with sparkling wine to make the ultimate party punch. Using real Champagne is an unnecessary extravagance when there is now such a variety of good, cheap sparkling wines from Spain and the New World on the market. Here are a few of our favourite sparklers:

Mimosa/Bellini/Tiziano

Mimosa, or Buck's Fizz, is a simple half and half mixture of Champagne and orange juice. The same drink made with peaches, or apricots is a Bellini; one made with red grapes is a Tiziano. A tip is to add the juice to the sparkling wine, which will reduce the over-frothing that tends to happen if you try it the other way round.

Champagne Cooler

1/2 small pineapple　　　　　*Sparkling wine*
1 lemon

Half fill a tall glass with ice. Juice the fruit and pour it over the ice, then top with sparkling wine.

Mango/Papaya Go-Go

Use either mango or papaya to make this unusual and startlingly good party fuel.

1 large, ripe mango or　　　　*1 big carrot*
*　papaya*　　　　　　　　　*Sparkling wine*
2 kiwi fruits

Remove the flesh from the mango, or peel and seed the papaya. Juice with the kiwi fruit and the carrot. Pour into a glass, stir and top with sparkling wine.

Sangria Real

Possibly the most popular summer party drink, Sangria, made with freshly extracted fruit juices mixed with red wine and given a sparkle with a splash of soda is an unbeatable way to relax on a hot day.

1 orange   *Red wine*
¹/₄ lemon   *Soda or sparkling spring water*
¹/₂ lime

Half fill a tall glass with ice and pour in a wineglass measure of red wine. Leaving the pith on the citrus fruits, juice them and pour over the red wine and enough soda or sparkling mineral water to fill the glass. Stir and drink through a straw.

MARGARITA TIME

Distilled from the fermented juice of an Agave cactus, tequila is most often drunk in the form of a Margarita. The classic Margarita is made with lime juice and Cointreau and served in a salt-rimmed glass, but frozen margaritas, like alcoholic slush puppies, have become ubiquitous. If you have a masticating juicer, like the Champion (see Resources. p. 147), you can make excellent frozen Margaritas simply by freezing the fruit before you put it through the juicer. If using a centrifugal extractor, freezing the fruit will reduce its juice yield, but will chill the drink.

Strawberry Margarita

If you can find a blood orange to make your Margarita, so much the better.

60ml (2 fl.oz) tequila   *1 orange*
12 frozen strawberries   *¹/₂ lime*

Measure the tequila into a glass. Juice the fruit in the order listed and pour over the tequila. Serve.

RUM-BASED DRINKS

Rum, made from molasses, is ideally suited to mixing with fruit juices. Bacardi – a blend of white rums from different countries – is the single biggest alcohol brand in the world, but many tropical islands produce their own brands of rum and each has its own characteristics although some, such as Wray & Nephew's overproof white rum are pretty hard to take unless heavily diluted. Experiment, also, with darker rums like Myers, Cockspur and even Bacardi Gold.

Piña Colada

The classic tropical cocktail. You can buy coconut cream in cans or, as a last resort, use one of the proprietary brands like Malibu, which is ready-mixed with rum.

2 spears of pineapple   *60ml (2 fl.oz) white rum*
3 large tablespoons (75ml)   *1 Maraschino cherry*
  coconut cream

Serve over crushed ice, garnished with a Maraschino cherry on top.

Rum Punch

Not a Planters' Punch, which is made with simple syrup and flavoured with lime and Angostura, but a long, exotic, slightly fizzy drink. Use the biggest, ripest mangoes you can lay your hands on.

1 mango   *60ml (2 fl.oz) dark rum*
1/2 lemon   *Soda water*
1 lime

Juice the mango and the citrus fruits, leaving on the white pith. Put some crushed ice into a glass and pour the rum over it. Pour in the fruit juices, stir, and top with a splash of soda.

Euphoria

Curaçao is a West Indian liquor made from bitter oranges (originally from the island of Curaçao) which is now available in a range of colours. The original remains best for this recipe.

1/2 pink grapefruit   *60ml (2 fl.oz) white rum*
1 spear pineapple   *15ml (1/2 fl.oz) Curaçao*

Measure the alcohol into a glass half-filled with crushed ice. Juice the grapefruit and pineapple and stir into the rum. The Curaçao can be floated on top of the drink or stirred into it.

VODKA-BASED DRINKS

Vodka is increasingly popular, particularly with people who don't like the taste of alcohol, because it has little or no flavour and can easily be disguised by mixing with fruit juices. We prefer to use a premium brand, such as Absolut, which is exceptionally pure and won't give you a hangover. When travelling, seek out the extra-strength, red label Absolut in duty-free shops.

Harvey Wallbanger

A screwdriver, vodka mixed with orange juice, is the most basic vodka cocktail. This is a more sophisticated variation, with the addition of a spoonful of Galliano, the spicy, herby Italian liquor that's sold in tall bottles, floated on top.

1 large, ripe orange　　　　　　　*1 tbsp of Galliano*
60ml (2 fl.oz) vodka

Measure the vodka into a glass, over ice. Juice the orange and mix it in. Gently float the Galliano on top.

Lucky Jim

A longer version of this classic variation of the Dry Martini, this recipe makes a light green, refreshing cocktail. A great aperitif, this recipe also works well with gin.

3cm section of cucumber　　　　*A splash of dry vermouth*
1 stalk of celery　　　　　　　　*(such as Noilly Prat)*
60ml (2 fl.oz) vodka

Put some ice cubes in the bottom of a tall glass and add a splash of vodka. Leave to stand while juicing the cucumber and celery. Add the juice and the vodka, stir and serve with a stalk of parsley to garnish.

Ultimate Bloody Mary

There must be more recipes for Bloody Mary than for any other mixed drink, but most are predicated on canned tomato juice and require wakening-up with a dash of sherry and a range of garnishes. This one uses raw juice and doesn't require such extraneous adornments, unless you are partial to them.

3 ripe tomatoes　　　　　　　*A dash of Tabasco, or*
1 stalk celery　　　　　　　　*Worcestershire Sauce*
5cm section of cucumber　　　*Salt and cayenne pepper*
60ml (2 fl.oz) vodka　　　　　*or grated horseradish*

Measure the vodka over ice. Juice the remaining ingredients, stir and serve with your choice of seasonings.

Resources

Green Foods

Lifestream spirulina and other good green products are available mail order from Xynergy Products, Lower Elsted, Midhurst, West Sussex GU29 0JT. Tel: 01730 813642. Fax: 01730 815109.

Chlorella is available in capsule form from Solgar Vitamins Ltd, who also do an excellent powdered green supplement Green & More. For your local stockist contact: Solgar Vitamins Ltd, Solgar House, Chiltern Commerce Centre, Ashridge Road, Chesham, Buckinghamshire HP5 2PY. Tel: 01494 791691. Fax: 01494 792729.

Wheat-grass juice in powdered form is available from Malcolm Simmonds Herbal Supplies, 3 Burton Villas, Hove, East Sussex BN3 6FN. Tel: 01273 202401.

Green Magma, the dried juice of young barley leaves, is available from good health food stores.

Herbs An excellent supplier of tinctures, fluid extracts, loose dried herbs and the Schoenenberger plant juices is Phyto Pharmaceuticals Ltd, 3 Kings Mill Way, Hermitage Lane, Mansfield, Nottinghamshire NG18 5ER. Tel: 01623 644334. Fax: 01623 657232. Minimum order £10.

Another good source is Malcolm Simmonds Herbal Supplies, 3 Burton Villas, Hove, East Sussex BN3 6FN. Tel: 01273 202401.

Herbs are also available from Solgar Vitamins Ltd, Solgar House, Chiltern Commerce Centre, Ashridge Road, Chesham, Buckinghamshire HP5 2PY. Tel: 01494 791691. Fax: 01494 792729.

Honey The Garvin Honey Company have a good selection of set and clear honeys from all over the world. These can be ordered from The Garvin Honey Company Ltd, Garvin House, 158 Twickenham Road, Isleworth, Middlesex TW7 7LD. Tel: 0181 560 7171.

The New Zealand Natural Food Company have a fine range of honey, including organic honey, in particular Manuka honey, known for its anti-bacterial effects. The New Zealand Natural Food Company Ltd, Hold Close, Highgate Wood, London N10 3HW. Tel: 0181 444 5660.

Linseeds or Flaxseeds Linusit Gold are vacuum-packed and very good. Grind the seeds in a coffee grinder and sprinkle on cereals, salads, in yoghurt or in drinks. Or put dry into a blender, grind them and pour on your fresh juice. Available from health food stores.

Other good linseeds can be bought from Higher Nature Limited, The Nutrition Centre, Burwash Common, East Sussex TN19 7LX. Tel: 01435 882880.

Linseed oil can be obtained in capsules from Biocare, 17 Pershore Road, Birmingham B30 3EE. Tel: 0121 433 3727.

Marigold Swiss Vegetable Bouillon Powder This instant broth based on vegetables and sea salt is available from health food stores or direct from Marigold Foods, Unit 10, St Pancras Commercial Centre, 63 Pratt Street, London NW1 0BY. Tel: 0171 267 7368. It comes in regular and low-salt forms. The low-salt form is excellent for making spirulina broth.

Organic Foods The Soils Association publishes a regularly-updated National Directory of Farm Shops and Box Schemes which costs £3, including postage, from The Organic Food & Farming Centre, 86 Colston Street, Bristol BS1 5BB.

Organic Meat Good quality organic beef, pork, bacon, lamb, chicken, a variety of types of sausage, and a selection of cheeses can be ordered from Eastbrook Farm Organic Meats, Bishopstone, Swindon, Wiltshire SN6 8PW. Tel: 01793 790460. Fax: 01793 791239. All goods are sent for next day delivery, vacuum-packed and chilled.

Sea Plants such as kelp, dulse, nori, kombu can be bought from Japanese grocers or macrobiotic health shops.

Soya Milk The best soya milk we have come across is called Bonsoy, and is available from good health food stores.

Special Juicing Equipment

The Champion Masticating Juicer
Veteran juicers wax lyrical about the virtues of the Champion, an indestructible, American juicer that some people claim

makes better juice than any centrifugal extractor can because its masticating action is more effective at 'trituration', the process of splitting open the fibres of the plant matter and liberating its nutrients in the form of juice. The Champion is basically a rotating cutter on a shaft, which expels dry pulp from its snout at one end as the juice is drained through a nozzle underneath.

Expensive, the Champion is guaranteed for five years and can well last a lifetime, easily repaying the investment in the long run. For details of your nearest stockist, or to buy a Champion by mail order, contact the distributor, Quality Health Products Inc, 922 Black Diamond Way, Lodi, California, CA 95240, USA.

The Vita-Mix Total Nutrition Centre

A turbo-charged, super-efficient blender with indestructible stainless steel blades and an extremely powerful motor, the TNC is dynamite! It's the only machine that is properly able to make the fibre-rich juices – the kind of molecular or *total*, juicing – discussed in Chapter Seven. It is also effective for making cereal grass juices (which should be strained before drinking to remove indigestible cellulose fibres). The TNC not only makes juice, but can also be used to make soups and ice cream. The Super TNC can even be used to mix wholegrain bread. These American machines are expensive, but owning one could change your life. Contact Vita-Mix in the USA for the name of a local distributor. Vita-Mix Corporation, 8615 Usher Road, Cleveland, OH 44138, USA. Tel: 001 216 235 4840.

SPROUTING

All you need to start your own indoor germinating 'factory' are a few old jars, some pure water, fresh seeds/grains/pulses, and an area of your kitchen or a windowsill which is not absolutely freezing.

Home-made sprouters

There are two main ways to sprout seeds – in jars and in seed trays. Jars are traditional, but we find seed trays easiest and best.

A simple, and cheap sprouter can be anything from a bucket to a polythene bag. The traditional sprouter is a wide-mouthed glass jar. The easiest and least fussy way to use them is to use open jars and to cover a row of them with a tea towel to prevent dust and insects from getting in.

Start here

- Put the seed/grain/pulse of your choice, for example mung, in a large sieve. Remember that most sprouts give a volume about eight times that of the dry matter. Remove any small stones, broken seeds or loose husks and rinse your sprouts well.
- Put the seeds in a jar and cover with about 10cm of pure water. Rinsing can be done in tap water, but the initial soak, where the seeds absorb a lot of water to set their enzymes in action, is best done in filtered or boiled and then cooled spring water, as the chlorine in tap water can inhibit germination – and is also not very good for you.
- Leave your sprouts to soak overnight.
- Pour off the soak-water. If none remains then you still have thirsty beans on your hands, so give them more water to absorb. The soak-water is good for watering houseplants. Some people like to use it in soups or drink it straight, but we find it extremely bitter. Also, the soak-water from some beans and grains contains phytates – nature's insecticides, which protect the vulnerable seeds in the soil from invasion by micro-organisms. These phytates interfere with certain biological functions in man including the absorption of many minerals (for example zinc, magnesium and calcium), and are therefore best avoided. The soak-water from wheat, however, known as 'rejuvelac', makes a wonderful liquid for preparing fermented cheese and is very good for you.
- Rinse the seeds by tipping them into a large sieve and rinsing them well before replacing them in the jar. Be sure that they are well drained as too much water may cause them to rot. Repeat this process morning and night for most sprouts. During a very hot spell they may need a midday rinse too.
- Return the sprouter to a reasonably warm place. This can be under the sink, in an airing cupboard or just in a corner not too far from a radiator. Sprouts grow fastest and best *without* light and in a temperature of about 21°C (70°F).

- After about 3–5 days your sprouts will be ready for a dose of chlorophyll, depending on what kind you are growing. Alfalfa thrive on a little sunlight after they've grown for two or three days but mung beans, fenugreek and lentils are best off without it. Place the sprouts in the sunshine – a sunny windowsill is ideal – and watch them develop little green leaves. Be sure that they are kept moist and that they don't get too hot and roast!

- After a few hours in the sun most sprouts are ready to be eaten. Optimum vitamin content occurs 50–96 hours after germination begins. They should be rinsed and eaten straight away or stored in the refrigerator in an airtight container or sealed polythene bag. Some people dislike the taste of seed hulls such as those that come with mung sprouts. To remove them simply place the sprouts in a bowl and cover with water. Stir the sprouts gently. The seed hulls will float to the top and can be skimmed off with your hand.

Make it big

Now for our favourite and simplified method using seed trays. Leslie finds that, with the great demand of her family for living foods, the jar method simply doesn't produce enough. Also, tray sprouts need only a splash of water each day. This is an extremely simple way to grow even very large quantities easily.

Take a few small seed trays (the kind gardeners use to grow seedlings, with fine holes in the bottom for drainage). When germinating very tiny seeds such as alfalfa you will need to line your seed tray with damp, plain white kitchen towels. Place the trays inside a larger tray to catch the water that drains from them. Soak the seeds/grains/pulses overnight, as in the jar method, then rinse them well and spread them a few layers deep in each of the trays. Spray the seeds with water (by putting them under the tap or by using a spray bottle) and leave in a warm place. Check the seeds each day and spray them again if they seem dry. If the seeds get too wet they will rot, so be careful not to overwater them. Larger seeds such as chickpeas, lentils and mung beans need to be gently turned over with your hand once a day to ensure that the seeds underneath are not suffocated. Alfalfa seeds can be simply sprinkled on damp paper towels and left alone and after four or five days will have grown into a thick green carpet. Don't forget to put alfalfa sprouts in some sunlight for a day or so to develop lots of chlorophyll. When the seeds are ready, harvest them, rinse them well in a sieve and put them in an airtight container or sealed polythene bag until you want them. To make the next batch, rinse the trays well and begin again.

Tips and tricks

Some sprouts are more difficult to grow than others, but usually if seeds fail to germinate it is because they are too old and no longer viable. It is always worth buying top-quality seeds because, after removing dead and broken seeds, and taking germinating failures into account, they work out better value than cheaper ones. Also try to avoid seeds treated with insecticide/ fungicide mixtures such as those which are sold in gardening shops and some nurseries. Health food shops and wholefood emporia are usually your best bet. At the latter you can buy seeds very cheaply for sprouting in bulk. It is fun to experiment with growing all kinds of sprouts from radish seeds to soya beans, but avoid plants whose greens are known to be poisonous such as the deadly nightshade family, potato and tomato seeds. Also avoid kidney beans, as they are poisonous raw.

Some of the easiest to begin with are alfalfa seeds, adzuki (aduki) beans, mung beans, lentils, fenugreek seeds, radish seeds, chickpeas and wheat. Others include sunflower seeds, pumpkin seeds, sesame seeds, buckwheat, flax, mint, red clover and triticale. These latter can sometimes be difficult to find or to sprout – the 'seeds' must be in their hulls and the nuts must be really fresh and undamaged. Good luck!

Variety	Soak Time	Dry Measure	Days to Harvest	Sprouting Tips
Alfalfa	Overnight	3 tbsp	4–5	Grow on wet paper towel – place in light for last 24 hrs
Chickpea	Up to 24 hours	2 cups	3–4	Needs long soak, renew water twice during soak
Fenugreek	Overnight	½ cup	3–5	Pungent flavour
Lentil	Overnight	1 cup	3–5	Earthy flavour
Mung	Overnight	¾ cup	3–5	Grow in the dark – place in light for last 24 hours

Sprouting Cereal Grasses

You will need:
A seed-tray (a kitchen tray will do)
Good organic potting compost
8–10 layers of newspaper
A sheet of plastic to cover the tray
Seed – hard red winter wheat or buckwheat, barley etc.

How to sprout:
1. Soak approximately 1 cup of seed for 12 hours in water (cover well), pour off the water and allow to drain for 12 hours.
2. Half-fill the seed-tray with compost (so that the compost comes half-way up the sides of the tray), level the surface and spray with a fine spray. Make sure you do not soak the compost.
3. Place the soaked seeds on the wet soil so that the seeds are evenly spread and not on top of each other.
4. Soak the newspaper thoroughly, cut to the size of the seed tray and cover the seeds. Place the plastic on top of the newspaper.
5. Leave the tray in a well-ventilated, not over-warm room for 3 days.
6. At the end of 3 days remove the plastic and newspaper and put the trays somewhere where they will get plenty of light – a sunny windowsill, for instance – and water once a day, making sure you do not soak the soil.
7. In about 5–8 days the plants should be 15–20cm (6–8"), high standing upright and nicely green. They are then ready to cut.
8. Cut the greens close to the soil with a sharp knife. They can be kept in the fridge in plastic bags for several days.

Cereal grasses can be grown all the year round wherever you live and regardless of whether you have a garden. Use organic seed, which should be available from good health food stores. Cereal grasses can only be juiced using a machine specifically designed for this purpose.

Alternatively they can be put into a powerful blender such as the Vita-Mix with 1/2 cup of raw fresh juice or spring water and blended for 10–20 seconds to pulverise them. Then you need to strain away the indigestible cellulose before serving.

Further Reading

Good Diet

The Bircher-Benner Health Guide, Ruth Kunz-Bircher, Unwin Paperbacks, London, 1981.

Nutrition for Vegetarians, Agatha Moody Thrash M.D. & Calvin L. Thrash M.D., Thrash Publications, Seale, Alabama, 1982.

Nutrition and Physical Degeneration, Weston A. Price, Price-Pottenger Nutritional Foundation, La Mesa, California, 1970.

The Prevention of Incurable Disease, M. Bircher-Benner, James Clarke & Co, Cambridge, 1981.

Nutrition Against Disease, R. Williams, Pitman Publishing Co., New York, 1971.

Life in the Twentieth Century, Richard Taska Jr., Omangod Press, Woodstock Valley, Connecticut, 1981.

Eating Your Way to Health, Ruth Bircher-Benner, Faber and Faber, London, 1961.

Dr Bircher-Benner's Way to Positive Health and Vitality 1867–1967, Verlag Bircher-Benner Erlenback, Zürich, Switzerland, 1967.

Diet and Salad Suggestions, N.W. Walker, Norwalk Press, Arizona, 1940.

Macrobiotic Diet, Michio & Aveline Kushi, Japan Publications, Tokyo and New York, 1993.

Subtle Energies in Foods

The Electromagnetic Energy in Foods, Dr Hazel Parcells, Par-X-Cell School of Scientific Nutrition, Albuquerque, New Mexico, 1974.

Man and Biologically Active Substances, I. I. Brekhman, Pergamon Press, Oxford, 1980.

The Phenomena of Life: A Radio-Electrical Interpretation, George Crile, W. W. Norton, New York, 1936.

A Cancer Therapy, Max Gerson, Totality Books, Del Mar, California, 1977.

What Is Life? and *Mind and Matter?*, Erwin Schrödinger, Cambridge University Press, 1980.

Food Science for All, M.O. Bircher-Benner, C.W. Daniel, London, 1928.

The Essene Science of Life, E.B. Szekely, International Biogenic Society, Cartago, Costa Rica, 1978.

Green Foods and Drinks

The Magic of Green Buckwheat, Kate Spencer, Romany Herb Products Limited, 1987.

Real Health Starts with Eating Light, Mitsuo Koda M.D., privately published.

The Wheatgrass Book, Ann Wigmore, Avery Publishing Group Inc, Wayne, New Jersey, 1985.

Cereal Grass, Ed., Ronald L. Seibold, M.S., Keats Publishing Inc, New Canaan, Connecticut, 1991.

Wheatgrass Juice, Betsey Russell Manning, Greensward Press, Calistoga, California, 1994.

Chlorella, Dr David Steenblock, Aging Research Institute, El Toro, California, 1987.

Why George Should Eat Broccoli, Paul A. Stitt, The Dougherty Company, Milwaukee, Wisconsin, 1990.

Nature's Healing Grasses, H.E. Kirchner, H.C. White Publications, Riverside, California, date unknown.

Wild Foods
Wild Food, Roger Phillips, Orbis Publishing, London, 1983.

Rejuvenation
Become Younger, N.W. Walker, D.Sc., Norwalk Press, Phoenix, Arizona, 1949.

The New Ageless Ageing, Leslie Kenton, Vermilion, London, 1995.

Therapeutic Use of Juice and Foods
Encyclopaedia of Healing Juices, John Heinerman, Parker Publishing Company, New York, 1994.

Total Juicing, Elaine LaLanne with Richard Beyno, Plume, Penguin Books, USA, 1992.

Food Power, George Schwartz, M.D., McGraw-Hill Book Company, New York, 1979.

Food Enzymes & Health
Enzymes & Enzyme Therapy, Anthony J. Cichoke, D.C., Keats Publishing Inc., New Canaan, Connecticut, 1994.

Enzyme Nutrition, Dr Edward Howell, Avery Publishing Group Inc., Wayne, New Jersey, 1985.

Enzymes The Foundation of Life, D.A Lopez, M.D., R.M. Williams, M.D., Ph.D., M. Miehlke, M.D., The Neville Press Inc., Charleston, S.C., 1994.

'A Turning Point in Nutritional Science', R. Bircher, reprint from *Lee Foundation for Nutritional Research*, No. 80, Milwaukee, Wisconsin.

The New Raw Energy, Leslie & Susannah Kenton, Vermilion, London, 1994.

Juices & Juicing
Raw Vegetable Juices, N.W. Walker, Jove/Harcourt Brace Jovanovich, New York, 1977.

Index

garlic, 29
gazpacho, 135
  pulp gazpacho, 117
Gerson, Dr Max, 7, 53
ginger, 29, 82
  ginger berry, 117
  ginger spice, 118
  gingeroo, 118
  ginger's best, 118
grapefruit, 37, 118
  citrusucculent, 115
grasses, cereal, 96–9
  hit the grass, 120
  sprouting, 152
green friend, 118
green goddess, 118
green vegetables, 61–2, 95–6,
  102
green wild, 119
green wow, 119
green zinger, 119

hair loss, 85–6
hangovers, 86
Harvey Wallbanger, 145
headaches, 45, 89–90
healing, 52
heart disease, 14, 16
hi mag, 119
hi NRG, 119
High Life, 57–71
hit the grass, 119
hormones, plant, 49, 50
hunger, 35, 70
hypochlorhydria, 82
hypoglycaemia, 88–9

immune system, 48, 75, 79
indole–3–carbinol, 52
insomnia, 87
insulin, 69, 88
iron, 74, 84
isoflavones, 48, 50

Juice Blitz, 30–45
juicers, 20–1, 67–8, 147

Kilsby, Dr Philip, 89
Kirchner, H.E., 99–100, 104
kiwi & grape with honeydew,
  140

lamb's quarter, 101
laxatives, 11–12, 59, 80
lemon, 37
  lemon zinger, 120
Leslie's cocktail, 120
lettuce, lazy, 120
Lifepower, 7
Linusit perfect, 120
low blood sugar, 88–9
lucky Jim, 145
lunch, 57–8, 70, 71
lymphatic system, 42, 55

magnesium, 77, 85
mangoes: fruit frappé, 117
  mango & peach smoothie,
    138
  mango go–go, 142
Margarita, 143
melon: black watermelon,
  114
  cantaloupe & carrot with a
    twist of lemon, 140
  cantaloupe & papaya
    smoothie, 139
  melon medley with berries,
    140
  merry belon, 36, 121
  potassium power, 123
menopause, 92
merry belon, 36, 121
migraine, 89–90
mimosa, 142
minerals, 46–7, 48
molecular juicing, 68
molybdenum, 74
mood swings, 45
MOP, 51–2
more raw NRG, 38–9, 121
muesli, 136
muffins, blueberry, 67

nettles, 100
neurotransmitters, 81
nitrosamines, 52

oats: live muesli, 136
obesity, 14
oestrogen, 48, 49, 50
omega–3 fatty acids, 50
orange seeds, 27